FOOD
FIELD  FORK

FOOD

FIELD TO FORK

How to Grow Sustainably, Shop Wisely,
Cook Nutritiously, and Eat Deliciously

To Gina —
Here's to your health.

Anita M. Kobuszewski

MS, RD

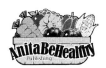

AnitaBeHealthy
Publishing

San Leandro, California

Cover Art & Illustration: Iqvinder P. Singh
Cover & Interior Design: Gary J. Withrow, Concierge Marketing, Inc.

ISBN: 978-0-9831165-0-9
Library of Congress Control Number: 2011911307

Kobuszewski, Anita, M. 1958-
    Food, field to fork : how to grow sustainably, shop wisely, cook nutritiously, and eat deliciously / Anita M. Kobuszewski.
        p. cm.
    Includes bibliographical references and index.
    1. Nutrition. 2. Cooking. 3. Recipes. 4. Wellness--health. 6. Aging. 7. Gardening and sustainability.
        I. Title.

AnitaBeHealthy Publishing
P.O. Box 211
San Leandro, CA 94577
www.AnitaBeHealthy.com

Printed in the United States of America
10 9 8 7 6 5 4 3 2 1

"Anita Kobuszewski has written Food, Field to Fork *with the same intellect, good humor and common sense that she uses in her work in educating people on nutrition. Anita's career as a dietician includes launching of the Wellness Program for the U.S. Navy medical department. I was the beneficiary of the implementation of that program.* Food, Field to Fork *is useful and the documentation with scientific sources contributes to its credibility."*

—Marilyn W. Schwartz, MLS, medical librarian,
retired director of libraries at Naval Medical Center, San Diego;
recipient of the Life Time Achievement Award
from the Medical Library Group of Southern California & Arizona, 2004

ACKNOWLEDGMENTS

It was by no mistake that the right people showed up in my life to teach me what I needed to learn at exactly the right times. I thank God for granting me the grace, good health and ability to complete this project. Next, I thank my teachers Mrs. Shull; David Lickteig; and Janice Dana, PhD, RD for always being kind and patient when I had a hard time grasping the subject matter. I am eternally grateful for the prayers and guidance of Sr. Julia Stegman, CSJ. She is definitely in Heaven smiling down on me now.

Special thanks go to my best friend, Marilyn Schwartz, MLS for her expert editing, research and writing skills that contributed to each draft of this manuscript. I am grateful for my cheerful intern, Christina De La Rosa, DTR for helping wherever needed. A very special thank you goes to my mentor and friend, Rita Mitchell, RD who contributed all the right feedback and technical guidance on the manuscript just in the nick of time. Rita, you are a genius. I personally thank my friend and neighbor, Jennifer Moran for serving as the bakery consultant for the recipe section of the book and Pat Booth, MS, RD for peer reviewing the initial manuscript. A thank you also goes to the great cooks whose recipes I have included in this book and the kind folks at the Dairy Council of California for providing the culinary related materials presented in Appendices F and G in the back of the book.

I am sincerely grateful to my editor, Sarah Harding Laidlaw, MS, RD, CDE for willingly taking on this project and for her expert advice, writing ability and patience. Finally, I thank Connie Evers, MS, RD who skillfully mentored me throughout this project and Joanie Greggains, Cindy Renshaw, and Dan Elliott for having faith in me no matter what.

Additionally, I thank the author, James Herriot, DVM for writing the most wonderful books about nature and science in the most uncomplicated manner from which I have tried my best to emulate his writing style in my book. To Garrison Keillor, America's modern day Mark Twain, for cutting to the chase the night he frankly told me that writing was a discipline and that I needed to just get busy writing.

Thanks goes to Iqvinder Singh, my faithful friend and gifted artist for designing the art for the cover of this book and to Nancy Crowe and David Lickteig for serving as my photographers. Additionally, I thank Lisa Pelto and Concierge Marketing, Inc. for being the best at all they do. I couldn't have completed this project without their expert guidance and follow through.

To my friends, neighbors, and family who willingly taste tested my recipes and supported me all along the way. You know who you are. I personally thank my friends Patty and Olga for serving as the appointed sounding boards for this project. I dedicate the long awaited release of the Opal Salad recipe to Michael Denten who has the most creative mind on the planet.

A heartfelt thank you to my Sea Dad, Lee Roach for helping me navigate life over the past 24 years. And finally, I acknowledge my deepest gratitude for the two loves of my life Toni Lee and Juliette Carmelina. Thanks for taking me on walks and making me focus on the important things in life like eating regularly, drinking plenty of water, getting good rest and never holding a grudge.

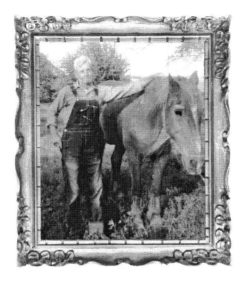

Charles Karber and his draft horse, Bob.

DEDICATION

This book is dedicated to my grandfather, Charles Karber. The blessing that got me through my childhood was the love I felt from and for my favorite human being, Grandpa Charlie. From Midwestern stock who originally settled in Wisconsin, he was born at the turn of the twentieth century on a farm in Kansas and raised a family of four during the Great Depression. A kind and gentle person, I recall him now with turquoise blue eyes and a full mop of silver and gray hair. His standard year round farmer uniform was overalls, with the white sleeves of long johns sticking out from under a work shirt. He'd wear the standard farming boots that lace up the front half calf high. Prince Albert pipe tobacco was his only vice.

CONTENTS

Bibliography 219

Appendices 239

Resource Section 253

Index 295

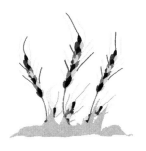

AMBER WAVES
OF GRAIN

Grandpa raised sorghum, wheat, milo and corn. My lineage is flooded with farmers and cattlemen from my mother's side. My ancestors plowed the fields with horses and sowed the earth with seeds. These Saxons planted and grew crops, grains, and produce for eating, selling, and bartering at market for cash and supplies. They raised chickens and cattle that in turn produced eggs, milk, cream, and meat. So, it was only natural that my mother would plant sprawling gardens every year producing mounds of luscious vegetables and fruits for her family. Some were eaten right away with the balance home canned and stored in the cellar to feed the family during the winter.

I grew up in the state known as the breadbasket of America, Kansas. Growing up in Kansas it would again naturally follow that I fell in love with the wholesome nuggets of grain and homegrown produce abundantly visible as far as the eye could see. From grains and cereals to produce it was all sweet, tasty, and nutritious to me. My grandpa's farmstead was surrounded by milo, wheat, and corn fields which he farmed and harvested with a team of horses. Even in the 1950s Grandpa tilled the fields of his farm with a plow drawn by his team of horses, Prince and Bob. Walking behind the plow rig he'd stride up and down the rows across the fields working the soil until the job was done.

Grandpa planted and harvested grains for his livestock, and when we were lucky, our family. In the summer months he'd pass along bushels of freshly harvested field corn and produce to our family of eight. (Yes, field corn is edible.) He was generous too, with the meat from the steers sent to slaughter, the eggs he gathered from the chickens he raised, and glorious tins of ice cream he bought from the local dairy delivery wagon, Grandpa was the most self-sufficient and sustainable farmer in my memory. His farmstead had an abundance of these foods as well as succulent walnuts and juicy mulberries. We all loved eating the wealth from nature Grandpa worked hard to provide.

· · ·

Oh the walnuts, yum! *Like most children I was oblivious to the fact that black walnuts were good for me. At the time, I just knew that walnuts tasted great and we could afford them because they were free. These walnuts were not like the store bought kind—they had a strong distinctive flavor unlike their more mild cousins, the English or Persian walnut. A walnut is ready to crack only after its husk turns from green and hard to a pitch blackish brown and softened husk. Once the husk was removed the shell needed to dry and eventually was ready to be cracked. Walnut cracking required the unsophisticated use of a hammer or rock to get to the tender, hearty nuts inside. The flavorful walnut meat inside each shell was worth the work. Served up on a cookie sheet the freshly cracked walnuts were picked out of the shell with a nail and would be eaten straight away. It was heavenly.*

Nutrition Facts: *Walnuts (Persian or English) contain omega-3 fatty acids credited with prevention of heart disease and stroke. Walnuts are flavorful, energy filled nuts containing cholesterol-free protein. The black walnut kernel is also high in protein and the unsaturated fatty acids that the body needs, but is unable to produce linoleic and linolenic acids.*

● ● ●

My grandfather set the gold standard for the virtues of kindness, generosity, gentleness, and sound advice. He'd give solicited advice and support to kindred farmers in the area. Once when times were lean he graciously had our family of eight move in with him. The stay lasted nearly a year and left me with many wonderful memories and life's lessons.

These true stories tell how I fell in love with the foods nature so unselfishly provided. Planting and harvesting a garden can seem daunting but not nearly the challenge as hitching your horses to a plow to turn the earth to plant and harvest food for a family for another season.

Follow the Yellow Brick Road

A weekly 'allowance' was nonexistent in my family. This was considered a type of socialism and not allowed. Without even knowing it existed, my father followed the United States Marine Corps credo of "Earned. Never given." Father ruled with an iron fist and this became an unspoken rule of our family.

Though I can't remember specific meals I ate while visiting my Grandpa, I remember his instilling the work ethic in me at an early age. My first job for pay was as the self-appointed dishwasher at Grandpa's kitchen sink. At about four or five years old, I would scoot one of the wooden chairs from the kitchen dinette set to the sink, hop up, and get busy. Grandpa always seemed to have a sink full of dirty dishes waiting for me to tackle. Each time I'd finish washing and drying the lot he would sneak me some coins as a reward. This was my first validation in life that work would provide me with feelings of accomplishment, love, and even some cash.

I'd save whatever money I would earn washing dishes, gathering pop bottles to sell at three cents each, detasseling corn, and babysitting to spend at the annual county fair and my hometown's "Days of '49." Oh, the glorious cotton candy, caramel apples, hamburgers, and Sloppy Joe's, I can still smell their drifting aroma beckoning me to this day! The county fairs each summer then and the farmer's markets or street fairs now remind me of Mom's words of constant practicality and self-restraint. Her last words to me before I'd leave for whatever adventure I was headed for were "Anita, don't waste your money. Make sure you at least get yourself something good to eat."

⬤ ⬤ ⬤

DETASSELING CORN: *A corn plant is detasseled to remove the tassel from the top of the corn stalk to stop it from pollinating nearby female plants. If a mature tassel was allowed to shoot up out the center of the corn stalk and spread its pollen—a creamy colored fertile dust eagerly bursting into the air—the nearby female corn plants would produce many ears of the same variety of corn on its stalk. Removing the pollen-producing top part of the plant so the plant cannot pollinate itself makes it rely on pollen from another variety of corn planted in the same field. This enables the plant to produce hybrid corn seed. To detassel, one would insert their thumb into the tight stalk's top, grip its immature tassel, and pull it straight up and out the stalk. Think of it as a church-approved form of natural family planning for corn. This stops "corn sex" and the pollination process. The seed company that hired us wanted us to prevent multiple eared stalks of corn as the ears would be smaller and less suitable for producing next year's crops.*

⬤ ⬤ ⬤

Another Day, Another Dollar

I still have a soft spot in my heart for grain because of my summer job detasseling corn in the fields about 30 miles from my hometown. At age 12, I was tall and muscular with auburn hair, tanned skin, and a face sprinkled with just the right amount of freckles. I believed that this job that paid $1.50 per hour would begin my trip to lifetime financial independence.

Corn grows well across America — from California to Florida especially in the Midwest where the summers are hot and sunny with ample rain and irrigation. The golden kernels of corn, when combined with beans, have the same protein value as beef. While grapes aren't blamed for alcoholism, neither should the corn be blamed for foods and beverages that when consumed in excess amounts contribute to obesity.

Eaten in its natural state, corn is a healthy food choice. Each plant, called a corn stalk, bears several ears of corn. Other names for corn are roasting ears, corn-on-the-cob, and simply corn. The freckled face girl that ate the corn has gone on to have a wonderful life.

Morning Muster

As the rest of the family slept, I was up at half-past three o'clock in the morning on hot, humid, and muggy July mornings. I had to meet the bus for the fields at Julie's Café by 4 a.m. Julie's Café, five minutes from home, was our town's only diner, open early every morning for the local coffee drinkers, farmers who had completed their early morning chores, and anyone needing a country breakfast to fuel their remaining day.

● ● ●

THE COUNTRY BREAKFAST: *To rural settlers in the 1800s and early 1900s, the 'country breakfast' was very hearty: potatoes and onions or pancakes, eggs, bacon or sausage, milk and coffee. Early hours and working in the outside elements burned off the calories of this high energy, cholesterol packed meal. Most Americans today cannot eat like this without plenty of regular exercise to stave off weight gain and elevated cholesterol levels that go hand in hand with it. Exercise was not called exercise then; it was called chores, work, and farming. Although the agriculture scene has changed, for the few remaining farmers providing food for millions, the country breakfast still remains.*

● ● ●

Just before 4 a.m., an ungodly hour for any elementary school child to be awake and functioning, with lunch sack in hand, I met up with other girls and boys awaiting the big, yellow bus. Down the steep hill of Main Street it would wheel, carrying a stout, mouthy foreman—a woman—and the bus driver. Miss Phyllis was a burly dame sent by the seed company to supervise our work. Miss Phyllis mustered us by last name. My name, "Kobuszewski" was always preceded with a pause or sigh because it was hard to pronounce. I learned at an early age that I had to lower the bar on folks being able or willing to pronounce my last name correctly. "Just call me, Anita," I spoke up to save from hearing my name butchered into yet another variation of "Kobuszewski." Correctly pronounced "co—bus—chef—ski," variations included anything from "co-boo-zoo-ski," "kru-boo-chef-ski" to "ko-bo-zal-niski."

Once accounted for we all piled into the bus. Again, Miss Phyllis hollered out another round of accounting. This time we numbered off. "1," "2," "3," and so on until the last child had shouted "!." She focused her critical eye onto her clipboard, double checking her attendance math.

With the count complete we were off to the fields. There was no waiting for latecomers.

We made ourselves comfortable on the elegant school bus, deep green plastic seats, some chattering or dozing. The thirty mile trip took about forty-five minutes down Highway 36 in the heart of corn country.

The standard uniform for the day included sturdy shoes, a long sleeved shirt, trousers, and a hat. Sunscreen wasn't a concern then; in fact, we hadn't even heard of sunscreen. As we stepped off the bus, Miss Phyllis gave each detasseler a large garbage bag with instructions to turn the bag bottom up and poke holes in appropriate locations for our head and arms. Voila, a raincoat was born to keep the heavy morning dew off our bodies. A silly get-up but effective and cheap. Our long sleeves kept the slender, scratchy corn leaves from irritating our arms.

Next, we lined up, one child to a corn row, and the detasseling process began. We made the tedious job as fun as we could under Miss Phyllis's eagle eye. Reach. Grip. Pull. Fling. Our goal was to get to the end of the row as soon as possible removing the single tassel from each plant. Miss Phyllis repeatedly hollered, "One tassel left behind will pollinate a whole field." We feared her wrath but secretly, I wanted to experiment to see if it was possible for one hot, steamy tassel to change the whole fertility cycle of an entire field of corn.

We flung the tassels up into the air as we picked. From afar it probably looked like someone was hunting for a lost set of keys or missing sock—or a needle in a haystack. The fling-fest continued until each row was finished. A brief pause and we were off again—either starting on a fresh row or maybe sent in to bail out a fellow detasseler who was not keeping up.

Lunch In the Field

I'm a natural-born eater. My favorite time of day has always been mealtime. Along with short water breaks, we would get ample time to eat lunch and rest. Each of us would bring a sack lunch filled with whatever would withstand the heat despite being kept in a large iced cooler. My sack lunch consisted of at least a couple sandwiches made with some sort of cheap lunch meat [ends meat] between slices of bread accompanied by loads of radishes and tomatoes from Mom's garden with an apple and banana for dessert.

● ● ●

ENDS MEAT: *Throughout my youth our family was financially strapped and I learned to love morsels of anything that came my way. My father, who eventually died of a massive heart attack, would buy the ends of unuseable loaves of luncheon meat such as salami or tube of liverwurst that the butcher could not sell to customers. He'd bring home this mystery package weekly and call it ends meat. I was probably thirty before I realized it wasn't "ends meet," meaning it helped meet our family food budget, it was "ends meat" named for the odds and ends of luncheon meat.*

● ● ●

Summertime is hot in the Midwest with temperatures in the high 90s to low 100s in the early afternoon. We'd stop work around 11:00 a.m. to get back to town on the bus by 1:00 p.m. My introduction to the all-American eight-hour workday began that summer. By the end of detasseling season I'd managed to not get fired for horsing around or for being late, *and* made enough money to live large during the fair and carnival season.

* * *

Nutrition Note: *Amongst the highest in fat, salt, and sodium-based preservatives is what is called luncheon meat such as bologna, olive loaf, and liverwurst. Very tasty and a source of protein this man-made sandwich stuffer is not a heart healthy choice of protein. With about 100 calories, 200-300 milligrams (mg) of sodium and about 7 grams of fat per ounce, this inexpensive protein can become quite expensive if it leads to heart disease, obesity, or other ills. Unlike in the 1960s, it's much easier to get a healthy sandwich today with the large variety of lean choices in the deli section and ample choices of whole grain breads at your local market.*

* * *

A Kitchen Baptism

About this same time, at age 12, I began taking an interest in helping my mother care for my grandmother. Grandma had a bad case of type 2 diabetes, often referred to as sugar diabetes back then. I got "baptized" into cooking, food, and the importance of good hygiene and cleanliness, as I learned to prepare food to meet Grandma's special needs. It felt good to keep her healthy with the proper foods and a healthy diet. I never forgot those feelings of satisfaction which probably first sparked my interest in nutrition and health.

Blessed and with a little luck, I eventually worked my way through high school and college. By the time I graduated from college I had met and married the "wrong guy." Nine years later I'd worked my way through graduate school and earned a degree in dietetics and foodservice management and shortly thereafter earned the registered dietitian (RD) credential. Yearning for unfulfilled adventure and challenge at 30 years of age I joined the United States Navy and set out to see the world—and see the world I have!

Somewhere along the way I grew to love mornings, have a respect for God and the abundance He provided our family, and appreciate the strong work ethic regularly modeled to me throughout my childhood. All these provided a perfect match for me to enjoy working in foodservice and dietetics as a dietitian. Now, over 30 years later I recognize the professions I chose were in Divine order and have provided me with a better life than I could have ever imagined.

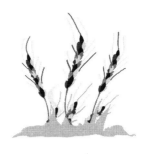

IT'S NOT COMPLICATED—
IT'S FOOD

Strive for balance in all things.

Food is fantastic. Eat healthy food often and shamelessly. I love to plant, harvest, cook, and eat. These are the reasons why I wrote this book and I am so glad I did. I am convinced that I ate my way through my youth and became a top notch athlete as a result of needing enough exercise to burn off the food I ate. This book is the written culmination of decades of working and living with food, nutrition, gardening, and cooking.

Whatever your reasons for reading this book, I hope you recognize that my approach is a practical approach to all things related to food and living. Take what you like and gently leave the rest.

Simplifying Food

I am not a saint. I do not live on celery sticks, rice cakes, and tofu, nor do I abstain from eating French fries, thick strawberry shakes or red meat. I've tried a variety of diets and potions to help me look and perform like an Olympic athlete gone super model. None have worked for the long term. Moderation isn't sexy. It does not sell diets or trick gadgets but it has been my salvation.

What you eat, how much you exercise, and how you handled what life tosses your way each day will determine your overall health for the long term. Simplify. Simplify. Simplify. Where nutrition is concerned, the key to healthy eating is to simplify all things related to food. Food selection, preparation, and eating don't need to be complicated. Good nutrition is a *one day at a time* deal. On a daily basis eat a variety of foods and fluids that are nutritious, taste good, and are beneficial to your health. Strive to:

- drink plenty of fluids, mostly water.

- eat more vegetables, fruits, whole grains, nuts and seeds, cooked and dried beans and peas.

- increase intake of seafood and fat-free and low-fat milk products.

- steer clear of foods with refined grains and added fats and sugars.

- eat fewer foods containing sodium and salt.

- be moderate in the consumption of alcohol or omit it completely.

The payoff is looking and feeling your best, both inside and out. Regardless of whom this country of immigrants votes into office as its president, *you* are the president of your body and mind. You have the freedom and the right, and most importantly, the responsibility to choose your nutritional destiny. Your nutritional destiny will eventually determine whether you are able to maximize your genetic destiny. The question is, does your *country* fall apart easily? Is your country up to fighting a war against infection, virus, aging or stress? If the answer is no then you can change your nutritional destiny now *one bite at a time*.

What Is Important

No beer, burger or beverage will transform you into a cool, sexy, smart and/or the envy of anybody, body. If you find one or several that can call me at 800-iam-nuts! You can actually think your way into feeling all these without shelling out an extra dime, lire, peso, yen or euro.

If you wonder what a civilization believes about food and health, observe residents in its rural areas. Without uttering a word you'll learn what is valued and eaten. These two observations will lead you to what chronic disease(s), a disease that persists for a long time, usually longer than three months, is likely to be prevalent. Imagine a culture that overindulges in food and drink, rarely engages in regular exercise and uses tobacco. Decades of medical research has proven that a population such as the one I describe would, without surprise, have a higher incidence of heart disease, obesity, hypertension, diabetes, and cancer. By no coincidence Americans suffer from all five of these chronic diseases. Nearly all are preventable or the onset can be delayed if healthy habits are established and adhered to daily.

Nutrition is much simpler than media and manufacturers would want you to believe. However, there is plenty of media-created hype, usually backed by advertising dollars, to confuse the average consumer. Don't get hooked into the hype from Internet, television, radio and print. These tactics are designed to get your attention, make you feel guilty, and this often only serves to scare and confuse the general public into purchasing something they think they need. Eating from a variety of foods in moderation isn't sexy, expensive, nor does it generate big advertising bucks and campaigns, but works like a charm.

When the chips are down people quickly get back to the basics. The reality of sound nutrition is most evident when a natural disaster strikes. After establishing or ensuring shelter and safe water, providing nutritious foods is the next critical element. If support donations include food you'd be mistaken to think barges or cargo planes stuffed with manufactured reduced fat, sugar-free, or light foods would be sent. The benefactors would send nutrient dense foods loaded with complex carbohydrates, plant-based proteins, and fat in the form of oils. Examples include protein fortified biscuits, rice, beans, powdered milk, oils and such.

Unfortunately the economic chips have been down in the U.S. lately and you may find yourself working three jobs with less free time. Be careful to not be seduced away from healthy eating for the sake of convenience especially when you're hungry, time pressed and have many mouths to feed. Now is the time to be disciplined and take care of yourself for life's long haul.

Sloooooooooow Doooooooooown

I admire the Slow Food movement for raising the healthy food awareness of many Americans. Joining the California 'why not' culture in my early thirties I first became exposed to the terms sustainable agriculture and Slow Food. Slow Food and sustainable agriculture are not interchangeable, but they are closely related. Slow Food is a global grassroots movement way of living and eating. Members link the pleasure of food with the commitment to community and the environment through good, clean food that is pleasurable and sustainable. I was impressed that the urbanites had once more renamed an old concept giving it a new spin and renewed sex appeal. In San Francisco I have experienced people devoting a whole weekend to Slow Food. A large group of folks gathered together to taste food prepared with Mother Nature, not convenience, in mind. Culinary artists showed off their talents and it afforded another opportunity for free speech to inspire others to change their habits related to food from the field to their forks and join the cause. Minus the large belt-buckled farmers and ranchers this event was similar to a Midwestern county fair food-judging competition. I say more power to them. There are numerous Slow Food communities through the US and internationally.

A Crossroads—To Change
or Not to Change

Are there food or nutrition related behaviors you want to change? Now is the time to start. Positive behavior change requires courage, commitment, action, and a willingness to not give up if you have a setback. In early 1983, behavioral researchers, James Prochaska and Carolo DiClemente developed a behavioral change model that assessed cigarette smokers willingness to make changes and tracked those changes across a scale of five stages of readiness. While their model focused on cigarette smokers, this same model is used today in many areas of health promotion and education.[1] It applies nicely to readiness to change related to improving eating habits. Where are you now on the ready-to-change scale? Are you in:

Precontemplation: My food intake is just dandy. I don't have a desire to make any changes because I eat what I like and like what I eat and it hasn't hurt me.

Contemplation: The idea of eating more produce really does sound pretty good. Maybe eating better will help me have more energy.

Preparation: I've put together a grocery list and have a plan to include more produce in my daily diet.

Action: Look at me, I've started including produce in my diet every day. From berries and broccoli to bananas and butternut squash, I'm sticking with it.

Maintenance: I've made eating five to nine servings of fruits and vegetables daily a permanent behavior change in my life. It's a lifestyle change I believe has helped me feel and look my best.[1]

Awareness is everything. Let's begin by changing how you think about food. If you're hungry for a certain food and you know it isn't in the who's who of healthy foods, ask yourself, "How will I feel 20 minutes after I eat this food? Will I feel good about it, guilty or indifferent?" If you think you will feel guilty, consider steering clear of that food for the moment until you can figure out what's going on in your head. Or, eat few morsels of the food and move on to a non-food activity and do not feel guilty about giving in to temptation. I've never had a client this technique didn't work for, including me.

Strive to eat foods that are as natural as possible and can be prepared with a minimum of effort or nutrient loss, or can be eaten raw. Produce is a great place to start. Try steaming vegetables or fruits, and then save the leftover liquid in the bottom of the pot for use later in a soup or sauce. This leftover liquid is chock-full of water-soluble vitamins and minerals which may help in disease prevention. Simplify. Focus on eating whole grains, vegetables and fruits. Plan to gather enough produce for three or four days worth of meals at a time. Choose simple ways to prepare them for your body and soul's nutritional benefit.

Are you terrified of learning to cook or just don't like to cook? You are not being asked to be a chef, but to consider making some small changes for the benefit of your health. Learn how to cook foods you like and prepare and eat these regularly. What you cook is good enough if it is what you like and even better if it is healthy. That *is* all that matters. While it is true you can destroy some nutrients during the cooking process, overcooking a food rarely completely destroys the goodness of your efforts. Give yourself some credit and grace for trying and remember that practice makes perfect. Sustain yourself as much and often as possible with locally grown basic foods or foods that you can grow comfortably in your own backyard.

Simply Healthy

Strive for balance in all things. Get back to the basics of simple and healthy eating. If you don't already, try cooking from scratch. Grow your own food if at all possible. Strive to build a firm but flexible foundation for good health and happiness through self discipline, determination, and making the most out of what you have. These qualities may not always be second nature but each one can be learned if you are a willing learner. Learning how to draw a balance in the quantity and quality of nutrients you consume daily is the key. Strive for balance physically, emotionally and spiritually. Remember to:

- be quiet, often.

- get good rest.

- consult your healthcare provider prior to beginning an exercise regimen.

- get at least 30 minutes of aerobic activity each day.

The pages in this book are my story about balancing food, gardening, cooking, and eating healthy. I encourage you to get your move on and enjoy your life just as I have—one bite, one step, one breath at a time.

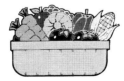

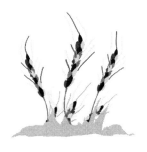

TWO

NUTRITION
AND BALANCE

"It is the position of the American Dietetic Association (ADA) that the total diet or overall pattern of food eaten is the most important focus of a healthful eating style. All foods can fit within this pattern, if consumed in moderation with appropriate portion size and combined with regular physical activity. The American Dietetic Association strives to communicate healthful eating messages to the public that emphasize a balance of foods, rather any one food or meal."[1]

ADA—July 2007

Strive for Progress—Not Perfection

I, too, believe all foods can fit into a healthy diet if consumed in moderation and coupled with regular exercise. From the Latin word *diaeta,* diet means a "way of living." It doesn't have as its root word "die" so get over the idea you'll have to die trying to eat healthy. You could eat a million marshmallows a day and that would be considered your diet. A diet is merely the food you eat in a 24-hour period. Your weight is what you weigh naked when you step on the scale, minus your cowboy boots and feed cap.

Nutrition doesn't start until food passes the lips. Accomplish this and eating healthy will fall into place. Eating a *balanced diet* means eating a variety of foods rich in nutrients including water, produce, grains, dairy, and lean proteins. If your favorite foods are fatty, salty or sugary, begin to scale back on how much of these you eat. Regular exercise and good rest help with the balancing act of striving for a healthy lifestyle.

Were the Hippies Right?

In the mid 1960s the term *vegetarian* seemed to be linked to tofu, grains and greens-only eating folks who were anti-establishment, long haired, tie dyed, sandal wearing hippie-types. About five decades later a poll done by the ADA, the largest group of food and nutrition experts in the world, indicated about 4.9 million Americans claimed to be vegetarian.[2]

Mainstream Americans seem to be getting a whiff of the health benefits offered in a vegetarian or plant-based diet. The term vegetarian has a variety of meanings depending on who you ask. Here are the latest definitions from the ADA:

- Vegan or strict vegetarian: plant-based foods only; no animal based foods including fish, chicken, meat, eggs, milk, cheese or other dairy products. Foods containing or made from animal derived products such as gelatin, are not allowed.

- Lacto-vegetarian: plant-based foods plus dairy products only excluding meat, fish, poultry and eggs.

- Ovo-lacto-vegetarian: plant-based foods plus egg and dairy products. Excludes meat, fish and poultry.

- Flexitarian: the newest category of plant-based diet similar to ovo-lacto-vegetarian with infrequent consumption of meat, fish and poultry.

Research has shown repeatedly that plant-based diet consumers, vegetarians, have lower rates of heart disease, high blood pressure, cancer, type 2 diabetes and obesity than folks who eat mostly animal-based foods.[2] Armed with this knowledge, let's begin to explore food and its benefits.

Eat What You Like— Like What You Eat

All foods, plus water, fit into at least one of the basic categories listed below. We, as a culture, are constantly trying to place a new spin on an old concept. The latest arrangement of the food groups released by the United States Department of Agriculture (USDA) replaces MyPyramid. The MyPlate Food Pattern, which uses a dinner plate plus a smaller container to define food groups and proportions, includes:

- Grains (breads, cereals, rice and pasta)

- Vegetables (fresh, frozen or low sodium canned)

- Fruits (fresh, frozen, canned in juice, or fruit juice)

- Dairy (milk, yogurt, cheese, and fortified soy beverages)

- Protein Foods (meat, poultry, fish, dry beans, eggs, and nuts)

Oils and empty calories (hard fats and added sugars) are absent from the breakdown of food categories this time around but oils are included in USDA Food Patterns. MyPlate emphasizes that the amount of food from each group on your plate should be 50% vegetables and fruits; the other half should be grains (at least half of these whole grains), and lean animal and plant proteins. Dairy is included in a smaller amount alongside each meal. Keeping this advice in mind, strive daily to eat the amounts of foods listed below that equal the proportions recommended by MyPlate. Make sure to include the foods *you like* from each food group.

Working our way from general guidance about what to eat, let's begin to examine more specifically what each food group has to offer as far as basic nutrients for your body every day.

Bread, cereals, pasta and other grains (5-8 servings): Provide B vitamins, iron, and other minerals. They are good sources of complex carbohydrates, whole grains, and fiber that fuel the body to optimal levels on a daily basis.

Vegetables (3-5 servings, about 2-3 cups): Provide beta-carotene (vitamin A) and vitamin C, fiber and complex carbohydrates that help with digestion and assist in the healing of cuts and wounds.

Fruits (2-4 servings, about 1½—2 cups): Provide beta-carotene (vitamin A) and vitamin C, fiber and complex carbohydrates that help with digestion, and provide potassium, and other minerals for healthy tissue metabolism and wound-healing, healthy gums, eyes and skin.

Milk, cheese, yogurt and fortified soy beverages (3 servings): Provide protein, calcium, and vitamin D for strong muscles, bones, and teeth.

Meat, poultry, fish, eggs, beans, nuts and seeds (2-3 servings or total of 5-6½ ounce equivalents): These supply protein, iron, B vitamins and other minerals for strong muscles and healthy blood.

Nutrition 101

The goal of this section is to inspire you to begin thinking about how to incorporate each nutrient group, by way of the foods you eat, into a healthy daily diet. Food provides nutrients, or chemicals in varying amounts that a body needs to live and grow. Simply put, our bodies cannot make most of these substances; therefore, they must be obtained from food. Nutrients are either micronutrients needed in small amounts, or macronutrients needed in larger quantities. Macronutrients are the majority of the diet, essential for growth and energy, and include carbohydrate, protein, fat, and water. All of the macronutrients provide calories in varying amounts with the exception of water. What are calories? *Calories* are a way to count how much energy a food contains. Energy you get from food helps you do the things you need to do each day—plus those things you do to have fun! Technically a calorie is a unit of energy or the amount of energy it takes to raise one gram of pure water one degree Celsius(°C).

It's an inescapable fact that nearly all the nutrients needed to sustain good health are found in the food and water. Generally, scientists and nutrition experts organize nutrients into six groups: carbohydrates, proteins, fats, water, vitamins and minerals. Additionally I have included functional foods or foods that, according to the American Dietetic Association, include whole foods and fortified, enriched, or enhanced foods which have potentially beneficial effects on health when consumed as part of a varied diet on a regular basis.[3] All nutrients, when consumed in moderate amounts, help the body function properly and maintain good health. Let's get this lesson started.

1. Carbohydrates

- Supply energy (4 calories per gram).

- Spare proteins to be used for growth and maintenance of body tissues rather than energy and are the body's *preferred primary energy source.*

- Provide fiber if the food is whole grain or is a fruit or vegetable that contains fiber.

Examples of food sources include complex carbohydrate such as fruits, breads, cereals, pasta, rice, and starchy vegetables including potatoes, corn, and lima beans. Simple carbohydrate foods include sugar, honey, syrup, candy, soft drinks, icings.[4]

It is worth noting that fiber, while not a nutrient, plays a vital role in digestion and disease prevention. Fiber provides bulk that helps food pass through the gut and helps prevent constipation. We will visit fiber and its friends later in this book.

● ● ●

WHAT ABOUT BOOZE?: *Technically alcohol, also called ethanol—hooch—firewater—nectar of the gods, contributes calories (7 per gram) to the diet but very little else nutritionally.*

● ● ●

2. Proteins

- Supply energy (4 calories per gram). If more is consumed than needed to build and repair body tissues these calories are used for energy or stored as body fat.

- Build and repair body tissues.

- Help antibodies fight infection.

Examples of food sources include meat, poultry, fish, eggs, milk, yogurt, cheese, dried beans and peas, nuts and nut butters.

3. Fats

- Supply the most concentrated source of energy (9 calories per gram).

- Carry fat-soluble vitamins A, D, E, and K.

- Provide a feeling of fullness and satisfaction since fats take longer to digest.

Examples of food sources include oils, shortening, butter, margarine, mayonnaise, salad dressings, cream, and sour cream. Less obvious sources the fats and oils are found in whole milk, fortified soy beverages, cheese, meat, fish, poultry, and nuts and seeds.

4. Water

- Is essential for life.

- Represents two-thirds of our body weight.

- Is part of every living cell.

- Is the means for all metabolic changes (digestion, absorption, and excretion).

- Is required for proper muscle and nervous systems function.

- Transports nutrients and all body substances.

- Helps maintain body temperature, especially cooling.

- Acts as a lubricant.

- Is required for the removal and excretion of waste.

- Helps curb the appetite.

Examples of food sources include drinking water, beverages, water in foods, and water released when carbohydrates, protein, and fats are metabolized by the body.

Wading in deeper on the subject, the body is made up mostly of water, about 60%. Blood, body fluids, muscle tissue, brain, and heart contain significant amounts of water.

Your body relies on fluid, mostly in the form of water, to stay alive. Since the body is composed mostly of fluids, it's important to drink plenty of fluids (mostly water) throughout the day to stay hydrated.[4] The body utilizes water as its own customized air conditioner as perspiration evaporates on the surface of the skin. All chemical and metabolic reactions that take place in your body happen in the presence of water. Water is recognized by all experts as the most affordable and easily absorbed type of fluid to consume. Water also promotes the feeling of fullness and helps keep the skin moist.

It's important to stay hydrated. Hydration is the act of drinking fluids to meet bodily needs. Dehydration occurs when there is an absence of those needed fluids. Signs of dehydration include fatigue, rapid or increased breathing, elevated body temperature and pulse, and flushed skin. If not remedied more severe symptoms may follow—eventually leading to death.[5]

How much fluid is enough for optimal body function? Research and opinions vary. First, whenever *fluid* is referenced here I mean a liquid that doesn't contain calories, caffeine, alcohol or added sugar. Second, bottled water is not a magic wand to good health. In fact, there is no measurable difference between bottled and tap water except for the expense.

After reviewing multiple references and guidelines on optimum fluid intake to stay well hydrated I've arrived at the following: the average healthy adult, not taking into account activity, should drink one cup of water or fluid for every 15 pounds of body weight per day to maintain good hydration or *at least eight cups per day.* For those who are physically active, additional fluid intake is required to make up for fluids lost as the body air conditions itself through perspiration (sweating). The actively exercising person should drink about 1½ cups of water for every 15 pounds of body weight. Depending on your current health, the climate where you live and how active you are adjust fluid intake accordingly.

● ● ●

Water Weight: *One gallon of water weighs about eight pounds. Fad diets often claim drastic weight loss in the first few days. This is usually due to water loss. The low carbohydrate, high protein diet requires extra fluid to help the body flush out excess toxins caused by normal protein metabolism through excretion via the kidneys, lungs, sweat, and feces. The scale will not tell the whole story if pounds are your only monitor for weight loss. A healthier gauge is a combination of how your clothes fit and a weekly glance at the scale.*

● ● ●

Don't like drinking plain water? Try adding these spunky fluid flavor enhancers to the water you drink or try on a new fluid ritual that'll keep you lubed and tuned one sip at a time.

- Add thinly sliced fresh lemon, cucumber, lime or orange slices.
- Add a teaspoon of your favorite fresh fruit juice.
- Try herbal teas which come in a variety of flavors and taste great iced.
- Add a couple of freshly crushed or bruised mint leaves.

Regardless your preference, drinking more water on a regular basis is a healthy habit.

● ● ●

THE GRAND CANYON HIKER: *Once upon a time there was a novice athlete who hiked roundtrip to the bottom of the Grand Canyon without carrying any plain water. She packed diet, decaffeinated soda pop instead. What? Yes, a total nut. She thought diet soda would be good enough to keep her hydrated. After all wasn't it decaffeinated? True, she did not die. True, she* *made the trip in good time. True, she was miserable. Thanks to the smarter hikers who customarily leave their partially full bottles behind for just such hikers as her, the last 30% of the hike was on smart hiker's water. Moral to the story is drink water.*

● ● ●

5. Vitamins

Vitamin C (Ascorbic Acid)

- Acts as an antioxidant protecting cells from damage by *free radicals.* Free radicals are compounds formed naturally when the body converts food into energy. Free radical exposure also takes place when humans are exposed to cigarette smoke, air pollution, and ultraviolet light from the sun.

- Helps the body make collagen, a protein that is often referred to as the glue that holds the body together. It connects and supports body tissue and internal organs.

- Helps the immune system work properly to protect the body against infections and disease.

- Improves the absorption of iron from plant-based foods in the diet.[6]

Examples of food sources include orange juice, grapefruit juice, peppers, papaya, grape juice, broccoli, strawberries, Brussels sprouts, oranges and citrus fruit, kohlrabi, sweet potatoes, melons, and tomatoes.[7]

Thiamin (vitamin B1)

- Helps body cells obtain energy from carbohydrates.

- Promotes good digestion and appetite.

- Helps maintain healthy nerves.[4]

Examples of food sources include enriched and whole-grain breads, cereals, rice, wheat flour and ready-to-eat cereals; pork including lean ham and pork chops; dried beans and peas; salmon, nuts, and oat bran.[7]

Riboflavin (vitamin B2)

- Helps body cells use oxygen to release energy from food.

- Helps keep eyes healthy and vision clear.

- Helps keep skin around the mouth and nose healthy.[4]

Examples of food sources include milk, liver, meat, poultry, fish, eggs, green leafy vegetables and enriched ready-to-eat cereals.[7]

Niacin (vitamin B3)

- Helps body cells use oxygen to release energy from food.

- Maintains health of the skin, tongue, digestive tract, and nervous system.

Examples of food sources include fish, liver, meat, poultry, peanuts and peanut butter, dried beans and dried peas, enriched and whole-grain breads and cereals.[4]

Folate (Folic Acid or Folacin)

- Also referred to as folic acid and folacin, folate is the natural form of the vitamin; folic acid is the synthetic form found in supplements and added to fortify foods; folacin also means folate.

- Helps produce and maintain new cells critical during periods of rapid cell division and growth such as infancy and pregnancy.

- Reduces the risk of neural tube birth defects.

- Helps the body produce normal red blood cells. The primary job of red blood cells is to move oxygen from the lungs to all the tissues in the body. Their secondary job is to move carbon dioxide from those tissues to the lungs where it is exhaled.

- Helps in the biochemical reactions of cells in the production of energy.[6]

Examples of food sources include enriched or fortified breads, cereals, flour, corn meal, pasta, rice and other grain products; legumes, spinach and greens, asparagus, beef liver, broccoli and artichokes.[7]

Pantothenic Acid (vitamin B5)

- Aids in the metabolism of fat.

- Aids in the formation of cholesterol and *hormones.* Hormones delicately work as messengers in the blood passing information from one cell to another telling each what to do next.

Examples of food sources include liver, meats, poultry, egg yolk, wheat germ, rice germ, tomato paste, sweet potatoes, oatmeal, and milk.[4]

Pyridoxine (vitamin B6)

- Helps maintain normal body growth.

- Helps the nervous and immune systems function efficiently.

- Helps to maintain healthy skin and red blood cells.

- Assists in the break down and metabolism of protein, carbohydrate, and fat from food.

- Helps maintain normal blood sugar levels in the body.[6]

Examples of food sources include chick-peas, fish (especially salmon, halibut and tuna), fortified ready-to-eat cereals, liver, milk, poultry, lean meats, buckwheat flour, potatoes, prune juice, and bananas.[7]

Biotin (vitamin B7)

- Helps break down and use carbohydrates, fats, and proteins in the body for food.

Examples of food sources include liver, kidney, egg yolk, vegetables and fruits (especially bananas, grapefruit, watermelon, and strawberries).[4]

Cyanocobalamin (vitamin B12 or cobalamins)

- Necessary for normal growth and development of the body.

- Helps keep nerves and blood cells of the body healthy and makes the genetic materials in all cells.

- Helps metabolize folate, promoting healthy red blood cells.

- Helps protect against pernicious anemia.[6] (Pernicious anemia results from the body's inability to absorb vitamin B12 due to a decreased intrinsic factor made by the stomach. Without enough vitamin B12, red blood cells don't divide normally and are too large. Without enough red blood cells to carry oxygen to body cells, you may feel fatigued. Pernicious anemia if left untreated, can damage the body's organs including the heart and brain.)

Examples of food sources include liver, poultry, fish and seafood (especially clams, oysters, crab, salmon, and sardines), meats, milk, eggs and fortified ready-to-eat cereals.[7]

Vitamin A (beta-carotene in certain foods converts into vitamin A once in the body)

- Maintains healthy vision and the ability to adjust to bright or dim light.

- Plays a vital role in bone growth, sexual reproduction, body cell division and function, and promotes growth of bones and teeth.

- Promotes healthy skin and linings of the eyes and the respiratory, urinary and digestive tracts.

- Helps body cells fight off infection more effectively and regulate the immune system; acts as an antioxidant protecting cells from damage by free radicals.[6]

Examples of food sources include liver; deep green, red, orange, and yellow fruits and vegetables; whole milk and fortified low-fat and nonfat milk; butter and fortified margarine, and enriched ready-to-eat cereals.[7]

Vitamin D

- Helps the body absorb calcium and build strong teeth and bones.
- Helps the body maintain good muscle, nerve and immune functions.[6]

The non-food source is sunlight which is why vitamin D is nicknamed the sunshine vitamin.

Examples of food sources include fatty fish (especially salmon, tuna, and mackerel), lean pork, vitamin D-fortified milk, fortified ready-to-eat cereal, and eggs.[7]

Vitamin E

- Helps body cells protect against infections and boost the immune system.
- Helps to widen blood vessels and keep blood from clotting inside them.
- Acts as an antioxidant protecting cells from damage by free radicals and promotes healthy skin.[6]

Examples of food sources include vegetable oils, nuts, tomato products, deep green leafy vegetables, fatty fish (especially swordfish, trout, salmon, and sardines), margarine, fortified ready-to-eat cereal, and eggs.[7]

Vitamin K

- Helps blood to clot so you don't bleed to death.

- Plays a role in bone formation.

Examples of food sources include green leafy vegetables, Brussels sprouts, broccoli, artichokes, asparagus, okra, dried plums, and green peas.[7]

6. Minerals

Calcium

- Needed for the building and maintenance of strong bones and teeth.

- Aids in muscle contraction and normal nerve functions.

- Helps blood vessels move blood throughout the body.

- Helps release of hormones and *enzymes* that affect almost every function in the body. Enzymes serve as catalysts in the body causing or accelerating necessary chemical reactions without themselves being affected.

Examples of food sources include milk, cheese, and yogurt; spinach and greens, legumes, canned sardines and salmon with edible soft bones; and foods fortified with calcium.[6]

Phosphorous

- Helps build strong bones and teeth.

- Aids in all phases of calcium metabolism.

Examples of food sources include milk and dairy products, fish and seafood, poultry, liver, grain products, legumes, nuts and seeds, meats, lima beans, and eggs.[7]

Magnesium

- Promotes steady heart rhythm, normal blood pressure and helps regulate blood sugar levels.

- Helps keep bones strong, maintain muscle and nerve function and supports a healthy immune system.[6]

Examples of food sources include spinach and deep green leafy vegetables, nuts and seeds, semi-sweet chocolate, dried beans and peas, whole grains, oat bran, meats, fish, milk and dairy foods and eggs.[7]

Sodium, Chloride, Potassium

These three work together to:

- Regulate the fluid levels in the body.

- Help regulate the nervous system.

- Help regulate muscle functions, including the heart.

Examples of food sources of sodium and chloride include table salt and processed and preserved foods. Potassium chloride is often found in salt substitutes, bacon, soy sauce and pretzels.[4] Potassium is found in citrus fruit, orange juice, tomato products, potatoes, grapefruit juice, green leafy vegetables, vegetables, milk and meats.[7]

Iron

- Helps regulate the growth and function of cells.

- Combines with protein in the blood to form hemoglobin.

Food source examples include soybeans, legumes, liver and other organ meats, spinach, ground beef, oysters, pork, enriched breads, flour and rice, and fortified cereals.[7]

● ● ●

MIGHTY IRON: *Abundant in nature, this essential trace mineral always works with a protein to carry oxygen in the red blood cells otherwise known as hemoglobin, from the lungs to other parts of the body, including the muscles. Iron is vital in maintaining optimal energy levels in the body. Iron is also a basic part of enzymes that help maintain good health. The type of iron found in animal based foods is called heme. The iron found in plants is called nonheme. Vitamin C, also known as ascorbic acid, when eaten with nonheme sources of iron, helps the body absorb nonheme iron food sources better.*[6]

● ● ●

Zinc

- Plays an important role in supporting protein and blood formation, immune function, and wound healing in the body.

- Helps support normal growth and development during pregnancy, childhood and adolescence.

- Vital for the senses of smell and taste to work properly.[6]

Examples of food sources include oysters, beef, crustaceans (crab, lobster and shrimp), canned baked beans, lamb, poultry, pork, fortified ready-to-eat cereals, and wheat germ.[7]

Copper

- Helps the body make hemoglobin and adequately use iron.[6]

Examples of food sources include liver, oysters, crustaceans, nuts and seeds, canned tomato products, beans, potatoes, lima beans, whole wheat grains, leafy green vegetables, prunes and semi-sweet chocolate.[7]

Manganese

- Necessary for bone formation in the body.[8]

Examples of food sources include pineapple, nuts, whole grains, oat bran, rice, spinach, and beans.[7]

Selenium

- Combines with proteins to protect body cells from damage by free radicals.

- Supports healthy immune system and thyroid functions.[6]

Examples of food sources include Brazil nuts, fish and crustaceans, poultry and organ meats, pork, grains, beef and dairy products.[7]

Chromium

- Maintains normal glucose uptake into body cells.

- Boosts the action of *insulin,* a hormone critical to the metabolism and storage of carbohydrate, fat, and protein in the body. Insulin is critical to the management of blood sugar.

Examples of food sources include meats, whole-grain products, fruits including apples, bananas, grape juice, orange juice; vegetables including broccoli, green beans, and potatoes.[6]

Iodine

- Essential to the thyroid gland in the production of the hormone, *thyroxine* for normal thyroid function.

Examples of food sources include seaweed, cod, iodized salt, yogurt and milk products, eggs, tuna and prunes.[6]

Fluoride

- Helps lower the risk and frequency of tooth decay.

Examples of sources include fluoridated drinking water, seafood, tea, fruits and vegetables grown in areas where the natural fluoride level in the water is high, and fluoridated toothpaste.[4]

● ● ●

FOOD FACT: *Legumes are edible seeds enclosed in pods. Examples are peanuts, peas, lima beans, soybeans, sweet clover, and carob beans.*

● ● ●

7. Functional Foods

Saving perhaps the best for last, let's review the emerging science surrounding foods that may have a health-promoting or disease fighting property termed *functional foods.* Trustworthy scientific research studies repeatedly show that functional foods have natural qualities that serve to delay or counterbalance some age-related diseases, promote good health, and may decrease the risk of or prevent certain diseases.[9-11] Vitamins, minerals, antioxidants, phytochemicals (or phytonutrients), probiotics, and prebiotics are all types of functional foods.[9]

- Foods or the contents of foods that may supply health benefit beyond the basic nutrients offered in the food itself.

- Examples are found in each food group. They may be naturally occurring or are functional because they have been fortified or enriched with a nutrient or food that has been found to bestow certain benefits. The substance added compliments the food it is added to.

Examples of food sources include certain fruits, vegetables, whole grains, dairy products, fish, tree nuts, seeds, oils, meats, fortified or enhanced foods and beverages, and some dietary supplements.[9] Plant sterols are natural components found in plants which can act as cholesterol-lowering agents and are often added to margarine.

Antioxidants

- Protect body cells against the damage done by free radicals.

- Helps repair the body against free radical tissue and cell damage.

- Vitamins A, C, and E, beta-carotene, selenium, lutein, and lycopene are natural antioxidants.

- Often naturally occurring in nature but may also be added as a component to other foods.

Examples of food sources include fruits and vegetables, nuts, grains, and some meats, poultry and fish. The body can make some antioxidants itself.[10]

Phytonutrients

- Organic nutrients found in plant-based foods.

- May decrease risk of chronic diseases such as diabetes, cancer, and cardiovascular disease.

- Accelerate healing and enhance the body's internal functions by supporting the immune system and promote bone and eye health.

- May reduce the risk of diseases related to premature aging.

- Often are naturally occurring in nature but may also be added as a component to other foods.

Examples of food sources include fruits, vegetables, whole grains and legumes. Usually the more colorful the fruit or vegetable the higher its phytonutrient content.[10]

Probiotics

- Found in foods or can be added to foods; may result in improved gastrointestinal (GI) tract function and better overall health.

- Live *microorganisms,* that are similar to the beneficial microorganisms normally found in your GI tract. Microorganisms are microscope life forms such as bacteria, yeasts and viruses.

- Also called good bacteria or friendly bacteria, probiotics may have a beneficial effect by helping balance the microflora in the body, improving GI function and overall immune function.[9,11]

Examples of food sources include active, live cultures Lactobacilli and Bifidobacteria found in certain yogurts and other fermented dairy products and various dietary supplements.[9]

Prebiotics

- Found in foods or added to foods that may result in improved GI function and better overall health.[9]

- Prebiotics are defined as nondigestible food ingredients that stimulate the growth or the activity of probiotics to produce one or several beneficial microorganisms in the human colon.[11]

- May improve overall digestive health and calcium absorption.

Examples of food sources include whole grains, bananas, onions, leeks, garlic, honey, artichokes, fortified foods, and certain dietary supplements.[9]

In general, functional foods appear to play an important role in a healthy lifestyle that includes regular physical activity and a balanced diet. Additional research is needed to further validate the benefits of functional foods.[9]

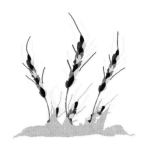

THREE

GRAND GRAINS AND FRIENDLY FIBER

Americans should choose fiber-rich carbohydrate foods such as whole grains, vegetables, fruits and cooked dry beans and peas as staples in the diet.[1]
—The Report of the Dietary Guidelines Advisory Committee on Dietary Guidelines for Americans, 2010—June 2010

Salute the Kernel

As the first food group mentioned in the song, *America the Beautiful*, grains must be special. As we know, making healthy food choices contributes directly to good health. Whole grains give more bang for the buck as they may help reduce the risk of chronic diseases such as diabetes, heart disease, high blood pressure, and cancer. Why? Whole grains are an important source of fiber, thiamin, riboflavin, niacin, folic acid, iron, selenium, zinc and magnesium.[2] The wealth of disease fighting nutrients contained in grain's tasty morsels help protect and defend against disease and provide nourishment to the body.

Of the food groups discussed in Chapter 2, four contain carbohydrate—grains and cereals, fruits, vegetables, and milk. The body chooses carbohydrates first for energy to sustain life. It's no small wonder that nature provides carbohydrates abundantly. While produce is covered in more depth later in the book, let's get busy focusing on grains and fiber.

Grains and Cereals

The grain and cereal group contains mostly carbohydrate based foods including wheat, oats, rice, barley, and corn. Foods made from grains are also included in this group; foods like bread, pasta, tortillas, breakfast cereal, and grits.

Grains are either classified as whole or refined. Whole grains include the whole kernel or grain, naturally providing more nutrition than refined grains. The edible whole grain is made up of three parts or layers: the bran (outermost, protective shell), the endosperm (middle, largest part of the grain), and the germ (innermost, smallest part). For a food or grain to earn the title of *whole grain* it must contain all three parts. The benefits of each include:

Bran: dietary fiber, B vitamins, and trace minerals.

Endosperm: mostly carbohydrate and some protein, vitamins, and minerals.

Germ: antioxidants, B vitamins, vitamin E, minerals, and protein.

Examples of whole grains include 100% whole wheat flour, cracked wheat also known as bulgur, oatmeal, brown rice, buckwheat, popcorn, and wild rice. Less well known whole grains are amaranth, millet, quinoa, sorghum, and triticale.[2]

Refined Grains

I believe that no single food is bad for you. Some foods are better for you than others. That's the case with refined grains. *All grains start out as whole grains.* To become refined, whole grains undergo a mechanical process called *milling* where the bran and germ are stripped from the grain leaving behind only the endosperm where the starch or carbohydrate is concentrated. The final product is a refined grain with a finer texture than whole grains, and providing a smoother feel like the texture of a doughnut, white rice, noodle or pasta. While milling extends the shelf life of foods, milling removes the fiber, B vitamins and iron. Refined grains include white flour, spaghetti, macaroni, saltine crackers, and white bread.

Thankfully, many refined grains have been *enriched.* The process of enrichment adds back in some of the B vitamins such as thiamin, niacin, folic acid, riboflavin, and iron lost during the milling process. The fiber part of the grain is not added back. When shopping for grains and cereals check the ingredients listed on refined grains paying special attention to ensure the word *enriched* is listed on the label. The ingredient label should state enriched wheat flour versus the label reading just wheat flour. This means the food contains B vitamins and iron because they have been added back in. Food made with plain wheat flour may lack both B vitamins and iron.[2]

Looks Can Be Deceiving

Brown bread isn't whole grain or whole wheat just because it's brown in color. What you may be buying is an unenriched loaf of refined white bread with molasses or a food coloring to make it look brown. Read the label. Ingredients are listed in order of predominance, with the ingredients present in the largest amount by volume or weight first, followed in descending order by those in smaller amounts.

By law the Food and Drug Administration (FDA) requires that for the term *whole grain* to be on a food label the food must contain 51% or more of whole grain by weight.[1] Look for the words *100% whole* on the product name which means all the grains in the food are whole grains. Anything short of this probably means the food was made from a combination of different kinds of grains or refined grains. Visit Appendix A for more on label reading.

Fortified and Enriched Foods

One last word on the topic of ingredients added back to foods. The terms *fortified* and/or enriched are often seen on food labels. In label jargon, fortified means nutrients are added to the food in amounts greater than naturally found in that food. Whole wheat bread that is protein fortified would indicate it has more protein than would normally be found in the bread. Milk is fortified with vitamin D that helps the body absorb phosphorus and calcium for bone health. Fruit juices are also sometimes fortified with calcium for bone health, but may also be loaded with sugar.[1]

You just learned that enriched foods have nutrients added that were originally lost during processing. Enrichment came about in an effort to prevent a deficiency by adding an important nutrient to a commonly consumed food. Processed grain products like bread, pasta, tortillas, and other foods made with enriched white flour are enriched with B vitamins lost in the processing of white flour.

Friendly Fiber

Do crabby, mean folk really need fiber more than psychotherapy? Wouldn't you agree that some of the crabbiest folks we know may feel better if they had more fiber in their diet? I think I'm right on both counts. Do all crabby folks suffer from chronic constipation? Is fiber the answer? Let's take a closer look at how fiber can *relieve* stress.

As early as the 5th century BC, the Greek philosopher, historian and father of medicine, Hippocrates praised the benefits of a diet high in dietary fiber and the effects fiber had on the body. Call it roughage or filler or bulk, since the beginning of time fiber has always played center stage to digestive health. Fiber has many health benefits and contains a wide variety of compounds that vary in their effects on the body. Research continues on the benefits and effects of fiber on the body.[3]

Fiber, found only in plant foods, is the part of plants the human digestive tract cannot digest. There are two types of fiber, fiber that is soluble in water and fiber that isn't. Therefore they are referred to as *soluble* and *insoluble* fiber. The term *dietary fiber* refers to both soluble and insoluble fiber. Depending on the kind of plant the fiber came from, the fiber type and quantity will vary.

Soluble fiber dissolves in the presence of water and becomes gummy or viscous like wallpaper paste. Frequently used to provide texture and consistency to low fat and nonfat foods, soluble fiber has been found to help lower blood cholesterol levels and regulate the body's use of glucose. Folks with high blood cholesterol or hypercholesterolemia and/ or diabetes have found soluble fiber to be a necessary and beneficial part of their daily food intake. A winning combination for heart health, a healthy body weight can also be achieved when you regularly eat foods lower in fat and cholesterol and higher in fiber. Examples of foods containing soluble fiber include barley, oats, peas, dried beans, and many fruits and vegetables including carrots, apples and broccoli.[4]

Insoluble fiber is sometimes referred to as *roughage.* It gives structure to the cell walls of plants and does not dissolve in liquid. However, insoluble fiber easily holds water. This feature allows insoluble fiber to add bulk and softness to your bowel movement, and helps prevent constipation by promoting regularity. Insoluble fiber helps move waste through the intestines. Because it gets a move on, fiber decreases the amount of time potentially harmful, toxic substances in food waste come in contact with the gut and its lining.[4]

Food sources containing insoluble fiber include:

- Wheat bran
- Whole wheat
- Corn bran
- Skins of fruits
- Root vegetables
- Many types of vegetables

Pushy Fiber

Fiber is useful to the body in many ways including providing bulk to help you feel full, preventing constipation, and possible chronic disease prevention. The old adage, "An apple a day keeps the doctor away" came from its fiber attributes. In summary, fiber has strong links with the prevention of a variety of chronic diseases and conditions including but not limited to the prevention of:

- Obesity
- Cardiovascular disease
- Type 2 diabetes mellitus
- Chronic diverticulosis
- Constipation

Eating adequate amounts of fiber may aid in decreasing the risk or possibly prevent these diseases and conditions.[5]

Meet Your Fiber Goal

According to the National Academy of Sciences' Institute of Medicine your goal for daily fiber intake should range from 21 to 38 grams per day depending on your age and gender. For children from the age of 3 to 20 years, the rule of the *age plus five* is applied. For example: a 10-year-old needs 15 grams of fiber (10 + 5 = 15) per day. This provides for a gradual increase of fiber as the child ages and takes into account the need for increased intake requirements once adulthood is reached.[5] Table 3.1 is a guide to use for people over age 20.

Table 3.1 Daily Recommended Total Dietary Fiber Intake

Gender	21—50 years	> 50 years*
Men	38 grams	30 grams
Women	25 grams	21 grams

*due to decreased food consumption
Source: Institute of Medicine, Food and Nutrition Board. *Dietary Reference Intakes: Energy, Carbohydrates, Fiber, Fatty Acids, Cholesterol, Protein and Amino Acids.* Available at: http://www.iom.edu/Reports/2002/Dietary-Reference-Intakes-for-Energy-Carbohydrate-Fiber-Fat-Fatty-Acids-Cholesterol-Protein-and-Amino-Acids.aspx. Published September 5, 2002. Accessed November 29, 2010.

Americans don't eat enough good sources of dietary fiber—fruits, vegetables, whole and high-fiber grain products, and legumes. Getting enough fiber helps to lower blood cholesterol levels and helps to normalize blood glucose and insulin levels for those with cardiovascular heart disease and type 2 diabetes.

Here's how to get enough fiber daily:

- Eat 5 to 9 servings of fruits and vegetables.

- Eat 5 to 8 servings of peas and beans, bread, cereal, rice or pasta. Focus on cereal grains with more than 5 grams of fiber per serving.

- Make sure to have at least half of the grains you eat be whole grains.

- Include nuts and seeds in moderation, as a part of your diet.

It bears repeating that eating fiber rich foods regularly helps maintain good digestive health. Fiber can absorb many times its weight in water and helps to bulk up the food waste, making it pass more easily through the digestive tract. An added benefit is the feeling of fullness that eating fiber gives. When trying to lose unwanted weight or just get better control of your appetite, make fiber your new friend named *Colonita*. She loves you already.

Rate Your Fiber Source

Research consistently shows that people who regularly consume adequate amounts of dietary fiber have less chronic disease. This same group of consumers gain the preventive attributes fiber affords.[5] Some foods contain more fiber than others. How do the foods you eat rate? Table 3.2 lists examples of fiber containing foods. Food labeled as high fiber or an *Excellent Source* of fiber contains 5 grams or more per serving. Foods considered a *Good Source* of fiber contains 2.5 to 4.9 grams of fiber per serving. Remember nutrients are always best consumed in the form of food.[1] Fiber, technically not a nutrient, is no exception.

Table 3.2 Estimated Dietary Fiber Content of Various Foods

Food	Portion	Fiber (g)
lentils	1 cup, boiled	15.6
soybeans	½ cup, roasted	15.2
Navy beans	½ cup, cooked	9.6
dates	5 whole, no seeds	8.0
raspberries	½ cup, raw	8.0
baked beans	½ cup, prepared	7.0
lima beans	½ cup, cooked	6.6
kidney beans	½ cup, cooked	6.5
refried beans	½ cup, traditional style	5.5
peas, green	1 cup, cooked	4.4
figs	5 whole, dried, uncooked	4.0
mixed vegetables	½ cup, frozen, cooked	4.0
pear	1 small, raw	4.6
almonds	1 ounce, dry roasted	3.3
blueberries	1 cup, raw	3.6
blackberries	½ cup, raw	3.8
sweet potato	1 medium, baked, skin	3.8
apple	1 small, raw	3.6
prune	5 whole, dried, pitted	3.5
apricots	½ cup, dried, sulfured	3.3
orange	1 medium, navel	3.1
papaya	1 small	2.7
banana	1 small	2.6
lychee	1 cup, raw	2.5

Source: US Department of Agriculture, Agricultural Research Service, Nutrient Data Laboratory, National Nutrient Database for Standard Reference, Release 23. Available at: http://www.ars.usda.gov/main/site_main.htm?modecode=12-35-45-00. October 1, 2010. Published October 1, 2010. Accessed November 29, 2010.

Easy Does It

Now that you're sold on increasing your daily fiber intake—take it slow. To avoid an internal tsunami (cramping, gas and bloating), increase your fiber intake gradually giving the bacteria in your gut time to adjust. Luckily, most high fiber foods are rich in minerals to make up for those absorbed by fiber as it moves through the gut. Easy does it on fiber pills and potions—these typically contain no nutrient value and may cause a mineral deficiency in people who already have poor nutritional intake. This is one more good reason to consume your daily requirement of nutrients in the foods you eat rather than from potions and pills.

*   *   *

FIBER TIP: *To help your gut get used to tolerating more fiber, increase the intake gradually. Instead of eating one cup of white rice, eat one-half cup white rice and one-half cup of brown rice mixed together. Then move toward eventually eating one cup of brown rice. The texture difference will help you ease into the increased fiber content. This technique can work for any food.*

*   *   *

Whole Grain and Fiberize Your Kitchen

To stock your kitchen with whole grains and fiber-containing foods from cupboard to refrigerator to freezer use this handy list to get started and be sure to make allowances for including your favorite foods. Remember—nutrition doesn't begin until the food passes your lips.

Vegetables and Fruits

- Fresh vegetables and fruits
- Plain canned and frozen vegetables and fruits
- Dried fruits (e.g. cranberries, apricots, plums, raisins)
- Preserves made with whole fruit (e.g. strawberry, raspberry, blueberry, blackberry)
- Frozen, canned or shelf-stable 100% juice with fiber added

Grain Products, Breads, Cereals, Pasta and Rice

- Whole wheat, rye, cornmeal, soy, and buckwheat flours
- Whole-grain and fortified breads, crackers, bagels, and 100% whole wheat or whole grain rolls
- Ready-to-eat fortified and whole-grain breakfast cereals such as Total™, All-Bran Complete Wheat Flakes™, Kashi Heart to Heart™
- Cooked cereals including quick-cooking whole-grains like oatmeal, muesli, quinoa
- Brown long-grain, brown short-grain, and wild rice
- Whole grain spaghetti, macaroni, fettuccini, other pastas, and couscous
- Corn and whole wheat tortillas
- Air popped or home popped popcorn, and lower fat microwave varieties.
- Wheat germ and bran
- Whole grains such as bulgur and quinoa

Legumes and Meat Substitutes

- Canned or dried legumes like garbanzo (chick peas), pinto, black, and lima beans; split peas, and black eyed peas (cowpeas)

- Dried legume mixes such as refried beans, hummus, falafel
- Soy protein such as tofu, soy bacon, sausage, yogurt, cheese, or flour
- Nut or seed spreads like peanut, almond, or sunflower seed butter
- Nuts including pecans, almonds, walnuts, cashews, hazelnuts
- Seeds such as flax seed, sesame, pumpkin, and sunflower seeds

Combination Foods

- Vegetable soups, beans, chili with beans, minestrone.
- Frozen entrees containing vegetables, grains, and beans.
- Canned or frozen vegetarian dishes such as chili or cheese lasagna or macaroni and cheese.[2,6]

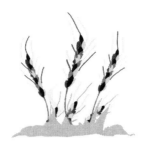

FOUR

KEEP IT LEAN—PROTEIN

*Plant sources of protein should be enjoyed often. They are
flavorful and typically high in fiber. With the exception of
nuts and seeds, plant-based proteins are low in fat.*
—Rita Mitchell, RD

T he Dietary Guidelines for Americans, 2010 (DGA 2010) were
released to Americans by the USDA and US Department of
Health and Human Services in January of 2011. These guidelines
are sound scientifically based guidance for healthy eating and are
updated every five years. This over 100 page research based document,
in its seventh edition, is summarized in Appendix B and includes
recommendations on healthy sources of protein to choose, among other
nutrition topics. Healthy protein source recommendations shifted from
mostly meat, poultry, and egg to a refreshing emphasis on an increase
intake of seafood, lean meat and poultry, fat free or low-fat milk and
milk products, eggs, beans and peas, soy products, and unsalted nuts
and seeds. The DGA 2010 went one step further recommending that
when Americans are faced with a choice between eating some meat,

poultry or seafood to choose seafood instead.[1] Let's learn about protein and the roles it plays in body function so you can decide for yourself.

Pumping Proteins

Protein is a nutrient at the center of life. From the frontier days when pioneers had to eat what was gathered or caught along the trail to cook over the bonfire, America's love for a thick, tender, juicy steak became signature of our culture. All of the organs, tissues and cells in your body contain protein. Your heart is a muscle and muscles are made of mostly protein. If grain is the staff of life then proteins are the building blocks, nerves, muscles, and blood of life.

Proteins and Amino Acids

Let's begin with what protein is made of and what it provides the body. Protein is made up of carbon, hydrogen, oxygen, nitrogen, and sometimes sulfur. The individual structural units or building blocks of proteins are called *amino acids (AA)*. Amino acids are the result of proteins broken down during digestion and catabolism. Catabolism is a normal body process where complex matter is broken down into simpler matter rendering energy. Regardless of its size or the composition of the AA that makes up a protein it is still called a protein.

Amino acids contribute to the following body functions:

- Build and repair body tissues
- Act as building blocks for hormones, enzymes, and vitamins
- Build and maintain muscles, bones, cartilage, skin and blood
- Maintain and support the immune system

- Vital to the proper functioning of the nervous system

- Help make red blood cells

- Aid in vision, blood clotting, and acid base balance

- Provide calories for essential body functions in the absence of sufficient calories from carbohydrate and/or fat.[2]

Abundantly found in nature in both animal and plant cells, AAs are essential to the diet of all mammals. Without AAs mammals would not survive.

There are about 20 different AAs that combine to make up protein. The human body is capable of making some of the AAs it needs but those it cannot construct must be obtained from dietary sources.[3] These are called *essential amino acids.*

Dietary protein is necessary for normal body function. It is an essential part of a healthy diet and the calories it provides are not a preferred, quick, or concentrated source of calories. Unlike carbohydrate or fat, protein is the body's last choice for energy. Similar to carbohydrate, protein contributes four calories per gram. All types of pure protein have the same amount of energy per gram: four calories. Meat, fish, poultry, eggs, dried beans, nuts, or tofu are equal when it comes to protein content per gram, but that is where the story line changes.

Protein sources are either *complete* and provide all the essential AAs needed for immediate use in the body or *incomplete,* missing one or more essential AAs. Animal protein such as meat, poultry, fish, milk, eggs and cheese, are considered complete proteins sources and the protein they contain has all essential AAs. Plant-based foods, grains, dry beans, peas, nuts and seeds, some vegetables, and tofu, while extremely healthy, are incomplete sources of protein.

Complementary Proteins

Nature devised a simple solution for incomplete proteins to become complete by creating what we term *complementary proteins.* Complementary proteins are two or more foods with incomplete protein sources that together supply adequate amounts of essential AAs to make a complete protein. These foods can be eaten in one meal or as several meals with a combination of vegetable-based proteins throughout the course of the day.

An example is peanut butter spread on a slice of whole grain bread. By itself, the plant-based protein peanut butter lacks the essential amino acid lysine that makes it a complete protein. But when combined with a food that contains lysine, such as whole grain bread, the body recognizes the combination as a complete protein just as if you had eaten a hamburger or piece of chicken that contained all essential AAs. Rice plus beans or corn plus beans are also examples of eating complementary proteins.

* * *

PROTEIN QUALITY: *Protein varies in its quality based on how easily the body can digest it and the AAs it contains. Animal sources such as meat, fish, milk and eggs are considered high-quality proteins. Plant proteins are incomplete and lower-quality, lacking essential AAs, but can combine with other sources to improve overall quality.*[3]

* * *

Proteins—Abundant Goodness

The nutrients in protein foods include the B vitamins niacin, thiamin, riboflavin, and B6, vitamin E, iron, zinc, and magnesium. Dairy products are included on the list of protein sources because the dairy food group is an outstanding and economical source of nutrients. Dairy foods including milk, cheese, cottage cheese, and yogurt also contain calcium and B-vitamins.[2]

Sources of Protein

Protein sources range from animal based to plant-based foods including:

- Meat: beef, ham, lamb, pork, veal, bison, rabbit, and venison.
- Fish: fin fish and shellfish.
- Poultry: chicken, duck, goose, turkey, and eggs.
- Dairy: milk, cheese, cottage cheese, and yogurt.
- Grains: wheat, rice, corn, and barley.
- Legumes: dry beans and peas, lentils, garbanzo beans, and soybeans.
- Foods made from legumes including those from soybeans such as fortified soy beverages, tofu, tempeh, and veggie burgers or other mixed dishes such as falafel or hummus made from chick peas (garbanzo beans).
- Nuts and seeds: peanuts, walnuts, sunflower seeds, pumpkin seeds (pepitas) including nut butters.[4]

Eating a complement of complete proteins is most important when the needs of the body are high for example during pregnancy, lactation and childhood.[3]

How Much Is Enough?

Choosing animal and plant proteins as part of the daily diet is vital to the overall health and maintenance of the body. The number of portions and serving sizes of protein recommended depends on one's age, sex, and physical activity level. Research indicates most Americans consume adequate amounts of protein. The current basic protein intake recommendations are:

Ages 2-13:   2 to 5 ounces, or equivalent each day.

Ages 14+:   5 to 6 ½ ounces, or equivalent each day.

These numbers apply to individuals who get 30 minutes or less of moderate activity beyond what is necessary for daily living. Protein needs increase slightly, by about an ounce per day, with consistent, moderate exercise. Note that the body naturally depends primarily on carbohydrate and then fat for calories—not protein. Protein is the body's very last source of energy during physical activity.[5]

To keep blood cholesterol at a healthy level, choose lean or low fat protein choices. Lean protein sources include some cuts of beef and pork, skinless poultry, fish, fat free milk or fat free or reduced fat cheeses, and game meats. Nuts and seeds, also contribute healthy doses of monounsaturated and polyunsaturated fats when eaten in moderation.[4]

Serving Size Sense

So how many ounces of plant protein are equal to one ounce of animal protein? One ounce of lean meat, fish or fish is *equivalent* to:

- 1/4 cup cooked dry beans
- 1 tablespoon of peanut butter
- ½ ounce of nuts or seeds
- ¼ cup tofu

Note this comparison takes into account the total calories, protein, vitamin and mineral content of the food. The exception to these portions would be when counting peanut butter or cooked dried beans using the lean meat exchange list for diabetes. This system counts 2 tablespoons of peanut butter or ½ cup of cooked dry beans as one serving of protein.

Keep it simple when you translate this into a serving size. Serving size refers to the typical portion of food listed on the nutrition label. It is found at the top of the Nutrition Facts panel and may vary from food to food.[4] A frankfurter may be a serving, but since it generally contains less than 10 grams of protein, it is not equivalent to a serving of say, one chicken thigh with about 21 grams of protein. Health professionals tie the recommended portion size to the amount that meets the daily requirements for a woman who eats 2000 calories and a man who eats 2200 calories. A serving of lean meat, fish or poultry is three ounces or the size of a deck of cards.

● ● ●

SMOKED-PICKLED-SALTED FACTS: *According to the American Cancer Society folks eating a diet high in smoked foods, salted meat and fish, and pickled vegetable are at greater risk of stomach cancer. Limit the amount of these you eat.[6]*

● ● ●

Vegetarian Vibe

Some advice for consumers of plant-based vegetarian diets was covered in Chapter 2. If you're striving to get all the protein you need from plants and do eat some milk and cheese, beware of overdoing it on the cheese with its hidden, and not so hidden, fat. More and more restaurants and grocery stores offer delightful vegetarian dishes that can be just as nutritious as those containing the traditional protein choices, but some may be high in fat if cheese is a main ingredient.[6] For more information, refer to the *resource section* that includes a section dedicated to *vegetarian eating.*

Peanut Butter, Baby

The go-anywhere food, peanut butter is tasty, economical, cholesterol-free and a good source of protein. With a serving size of 2 tablespoons it provides about 190 calories, 7 grams of protein and 16 grams of heart healthy fat. To slightly decrease the fat in natural peanut butter, pour off the oil that gathers at the top. You can easily make your own using a food processor. Just dump in the skinless peanuts (legumes) and grind them to the consistency you'd like.

*   *   *

BLENDER BLUNDERS: *When making homemade peanut butter with raw peanuts, be sure to use a food processor, not a blender. Blenders aren't made to withstand the drag peanuts place on the blades as it chops the nuts.*

*   *   *

A wonderfully convenient food to take along when you travel, peanut butter is easily spread on whole grain crackers, whole wheat bread, celery, carrots, bananas, apples and more. Topping your whole grain toast with peanut butter instead of butter can add protein and great flavor to a healthy breakfast. Don't leave home without it packed in your suitcase or seabag.

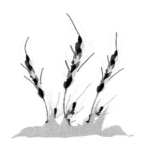

FIVE

FATS

Consume less than 10% of calories from saturated fatty acids by replacing them with monounsaturated and polyunsaturated fatty acids.[1]
—Dietary Guidelines for Americans, 2010

Not Naughty—FAT

Fat isn't a bad word or a bad food. Breasts and buttocks are made mostly of fat. Given America's love for both, fat can't be all bad. You sit on fat (your buttocks), body fat protects your vital organs from injury in times of accidents, helps keep you warm, and protects your bones from trauma if hit. Some folks even buy fake fat to change the shape of their body contour.

Fat is made up of fatty acids composed of oxygen, hydrogen, and carbon. Fat is a member of the lipid family, a group of oils, triglycerides, and waxes, which are oily to the touch and not water-soluble. Like links in a chain come together to make a fence, fatty acids do the same to create fat. Cholesterol is also a member of this lipid family.

Fats

Fat is fat is fat. Dietary fat is necessary for normal body function. Fat found in food is a beneficial part of a healthy diet and is a potent source of energy or calories as compared to carbohydrate, and protein. Protein and carbohydrate contain less than half the energy with four calories per gram to fat's nine. All types of fat have the same amount of energy per gram whether it is lard, margarine, oil, butter, or bacon fat. They are all equals when it comes to calories, but that is where the similarities end.

Fat Functions

A slippery topic, the best way to learn about fat is to start by describing how fat functions in the body. Visualize equal amounts of water and fat, whether in solid or liquid state. If you try to mix them, they don't mix. Regardless of the amount of either, the fat will always separate from the water. In your blood the watery component and fat don't mix, either. In your blood the fat is commonly referred to as *cholesterol,* a wax-like substance and member of the lipid family. Protein wraps around these lipids like a cocoon to carry it where it needs to go; the lipid-protein package is referred to as *lipoprotein.* Just as there are good and evil in the world so is true for lipoproteins. The *good* are the high density lipoproteins or *HDLs* (remember happy and little) while the *bad* are the low density lipoproteins or *LDLs* (think lousy and large). HDL cholesterol helps to prevent heart disease, and reduce the risk of cancer and diabetes; elevated levels of LDL cholesterol increase the risk for these diseases.

Fat also carries the four fat-soluble vitamins A, D, E, and K to where the body needs them. For a refresher on these vitamins see Chapter 2. Additionally, fat is a building block for vitamin D, bile salts, and some types of hormones. Dietary fat contributes flavor and texture to foods and helps us feel like we've had enough to eat, also called satiety.

The DGA 2010 recommends we eat fewer foods with added solid fats for better health and disease prevention. Specific recommendations include reducing dietary cholesterol intake to less than 300 mg daily, reducing saturated fat intake to 7-10% of total calories, and when choosing dietary fat, to consume more monounsaturated and polyunsaturated fats.[1]

Types and Sources of Dietary Fat

Nature produces fat in three varieties: unsaturated, saturated, and trans fatty acids. Within the unsaturated group are monounsaturated and polyunsaturated fats. Saturated fats are hard and retain their shape at room temperature. Trans fats are found in small amounts in milk and beef, however the majority of the American intake is now from hydrogenated oils. A food may contain one, two or all three types of these fats as well as cholesterol. It's important to learn how each one can affect your health.

Monounsaturated fats are found primarily in the oil of certain plants and their seeds and are naturally liquid at room temperature. Reducing saturated fat intake to less than 10% of daily calories and replacing it with monounsaturated and/or polyunsaturated fat is associated with reduced blood cholesterol levels thereby decreasing the risk of cardiovascular disease.[1] Foods that are high in monounsaturated fats include canola oil, olive oil, peanut oil, nuts, and avocados.

Polyunsaturated fats are also found in the oil of certain plants and their seeds and are naturally liquid at room temperature. These fats can also help decrease heart disease risk by lowering LDL cholesterol in the blood. Foods high in polyunsaturated fats include corn, sunflower, safflower, and soybean oils. To decrease the fat in your diet, choose fewer foods with fat. To achieve a healthy balance of fats in your diet, choose foods with monounsaturated and polyunsaturated fats, limit saturated fats, and avoid trans fats whenever possible.

Not Just Another Fish Story

Omega-3 fatty acids (omega-3s) are a type of polyunsaturated fat found in a variety of foods. Omega-3s are most commonly associated with fatty fish such as salmon, mackerel, sardines, lake trout, herring, albacore tuna, and halibut. The oils from these fish named eicosapentaenoic acid or EPA, and docosahexaenoic acid or DHA are also available as dietary supplements for those persons whose diets fall short in these important fats. Non-animal sources of omega-3s include canola oil, walnuts, soybeans, tofu and flaxseed which are high in the oil called alpha-linolenic acid or ALA. Alpha-linolenic acid is somewhat different than EPA and DHA so it must be converted into one of these two forms to be used by the body. Research has shown omega-3s may reduce the risk of heart disease and stroke by inhibiting blood platelets from clumping together thereby reducing the risk of clot formation and heart attack or stroke.

Additionally, omega-3 fatty acids have been shown to reduce the level of *triglycerides* in the blood. Triglycerides are fats found in body fat and the bloodstream. Elevated triglycerides can contribute to the narrowing and hardening of arteries leading to heart disease.

Research suggests that omega-3s may also reduce the risk of other chronic diseases. Studies continue on the positive role of omega-3s in depression, Alzheimer's Disease, inflammatory disease and the immune system.[2] More research and stronger evidence are needed to validate its health benefits. We'll revisit the seafood and omega-3 connection at the end of this chapter.

Saturated Fats

Saturated fats are easily spotted as being solid at room temperature. While mostly derived from animal sources, saturated fats are also found in some plants. Opposite of the monounsaturated and polyunsaturated fats, saturated fats can increase risk of heart disease by increasing the LDL cholesterol in the blood. Foods high in saturated fats include animal fat, lard, butter, whole milk dairy products, coconut oil, palm oil, cocoa butter, and many baked goods made with these types of fat. Don't forget foods containing saturated fat that we sometimes overlook such as grain-based desserts (cake, cookies, pie, cobbler, sweet rolls, pastries, and donuts) and highly processed foods including pizza, regular cheese, sausage, franks, ribs, bacon, and fried potatoes.[1]

Trans Fats—Mostly Man-Made

Nature doesn't hydrogenate fats. A trans fat, also termed *industrial trans fat,* is a type of man-made fat created by a process known as *hydrogenation.* Hydrogenation occurs by heating liquid vegetable oils in the presence of hydrogen gas thereby modifying the fat to become solid at room temperature. Like putting lipstick on a pig, we've eventually learned that the disguise didn't work.

Making liquid oils into solid fats was created for the purpose of selling sticks of margarine, extending product shelf life of snack foods, and making snacks foods maintain their flavor longer. These foods aren't ideal for good health. Industrial trans fats have been shown to increase heart disease and diabetes risk by increasing the LDL cholesterol in the blood. Throughout this manuscript whenever I refer to trans fat I am referring to the man-made industrial trans fat.

Nature does produce a small amount of trans fat in the rumen or stomach of grazing animals like cattle. For sake of clarity, this is a *natural trans fat.* Hence a small amount of natural trans fats are found in lamb, beef, pork, butter and milk. Trans fatty acids from natural sources are not problematic because with each one comes an abundance of other nutritional benefits that the man-made trans fat containing foods lack.

According to the FDA, the average American consumes 5.8 grams of trans fat per day (2.6% of total daily calories).[3] Consumer research has shown that of the total trans fat Americans consumed about 79% came from highly processed foods such as cakes, cookies, crackers, pies, bread, margarine, French fries, potato chips, corn chips, microwave popcorn, and household shortening. The remaining 21% came from naturally occurring trans fats in foods from animal sources.[4]

Since 2006, when the FDA made declaring trans fats on Nutrition Facts labels mandatory, it has become easier for consumers to spot these unhealthy choices on the grocery store shelf. That said, manufacturer's have eliminated a great deal of the trans fats in processed foods they make. The DGA 2010 findings include a recommendation to avoid hydrogenated sources of trans fats leaving small amounts from natural sources of trans fats as the dietary choice.[1]

Cholesterol

Cholesterol is found in the tissue of all living things with a heartbeat. Cholesterol is a wax-like substance found in the body and makes up cell membranes of all animals. It is essential for making steroids, vitamin D and bile salts that aid in the digestion of dietary fat. Plants have never contained cholesterol but their fats, particularly if saturated, can promote cholesterol production in the body.

Beef, eggs, poultry, and milk all contain cholesterol because they come from a living breathing animal with a heartbeat. Sources of cholesterol include egg yolks, meat, butter, whole or 2% milk, liver and other organ meats, and foods made with any of these. Many fats that are solid at room temperature such as butter or lard contain some cholesterol. The few exceptions to this rule are hydrogenated vegetable fat, coconut and tropical palm oils.

Plant-based foods, in their natural unprocessed form have never and will never contain cholesterol. Examples include corn oil, avocados, nuts and their nut spreads and olive oil because they come from plant sources.

HDLs and LDLs are types of serum or blood cholesterol. HDLs contain a tiny amount of cholesterol wrapped in protein for transport in the blood while LDLs contain mostly cholesterol with just enough protein to transport itself in the blood. HDL cholesterol is often referred to as the blood's *Drano*™ helping to bind to bad cholesterol, transporting it into the liver and then out of the body through the colon.

So What's the Big Fat Deal?

Overweight, obesity, and blood fat and disease risk go hand in hand. The big deal is we can greatly influence the risk of heart disease, cancer, and diabetes by paying attention to what and how much we eat and other lifestyle habits. While some risk factors can't be changed such as age, gender, and genetics (your parents), other risk factors can be modified or avoided. Modifiable risk factors include high blood pressure, elevated cholesterol, cigarette smoking, obesity, diabetes and blood sugar management, exercise, and low blood HDL levels.

A diet high in trans fat and saturated fat can raise blood cholesterol levels increasing the probability of having a heart attack, stroke, cancer, and type 2 diabetes. By modifying the kind and amount of fat in your diet you can reduce or modify these risks.

Are You at Risk?

The National Institute of Health (NIH) National Heart, Lung and Blood Institute (NHLBI) provides authoritative guidelines for dietary fat and sodium intake. Being *at risk* for a specific disease means you have more chances of developing that disease because of your behaviors, genetics, or both. The NHLBI's dietary recommendations for heart health known as the *Therapeutic Lifestyle Change (TLC)* program advises that individuals at risk for heart disease or who already have heart disease, limit their dietary fat intake to 25% to 35% of total calories per day. Saturated fat should represent less than 7% of total calories consumed daily. Finally, the NHLBI recommends no more than 200 mg of dietary cholesterol per day.

The TLC recommendations include diet, physical activity, maintaining a healthy blood pressure, and weight control under the care of a healthcare provider to help lower LDL levels in the blood. The NHLBI also addresses sodium and calorie needs to help individuals with high blood pressure or overweight concerns discussed later in Chapter 8. For those not at risk, or with one or none of the major risk factors the TLC is still an excellent lifestyle and eating plan to follow.[5]

The major risk factors that affect LDL levels include:

- Cigarette smoking.

- High blood pressure = 140/90 mmHg or higher or on blood pressure medication.

- Low HDL blood cholesterol = less than 40 mg/dl.

- Family history of early heart disease = heart disease in father or brother before age 55; heart disease in mother or sister before 65.

- Age = men 45 years or older; women 55 years or older.[5]

For those with one or no risk factors, prudent guidelines include the TLC guidelines with a modified goal for dietary cholesterol intake of 300 mg or less daily.[1] Use this chart to make healthy fat choices every day.

MONO-UNSATURATED FATS (HEALTHY)	POLY-UNSATURATED FATS (HEALTHY)	SATURATED FATS (LEAST HEALTHY)
Canola oil Olive oil Peanut oil Almond oil Avocado oil	Corn oil Margarine, tub-type* Safflower oil Soybean oil Sunflower oil Flaxseed oil Walnut oil Sesame oil	Butter ** Vegetable shortening Lard** Bacon drippings** Stick Margarine Coconut oil

*made with PUFA (polyunsaturated fatty acids), **contains cholesterol

Fat Math

When it comes to eating and controlling fat intake it's handy to know how to figure out how calories relate to percentages and grams of fat in your diet. See Table 5.1 for an easy guide to translate fat grams into calories and percentage of fat in a diet. Remember from Chapter 2 that one gram of fat equals 9 calories. If you eat about 1800 calories per day and want 25% of those calories to come from fat multiply total calories by 25%, or 0.25. The result is 450 calories, 50 grams, or 10 teaspoons that can come from fat.

Table 5.1 Percentage of Fat Related to Calories Consumed Daily

Total calories	25% cal from fat	Fat* grams	Fat in ~tsp	30% cal from fat	Fat* grams	Fat in ~tsp
1800	450 cal.	50	10	540 cal.	60	12
2200	550 cal.	61	12	660 cal.	73	14
2400	600 cal.	67	13	720 cal.	80	16

*Total fat calories include all the fat that is found naturally in food and fat or added to foods in cooking.

Naturally occurring fats are found in meat, fish, poultry, milk and dairy, cheese, oil, nuts, butter, grains and cereals, and avocado. Processed foods contain fats as well, but they are usually added to enhance flavor. Cooking with oil and adding butter or margarine to foods are also sources of fats and fat calories.

Healthy Fats in Seafood

While some of the heart protecting omega-3 fats discussed earlier are found in nuts and seeds, the most concentrated source is found in seafood. Fatty fish are rich sources of omega-3 fatty acids. Salmon, lake trout, mackerel, herring, sardines, and albacore tuna are among those fish highest in omega-3 fatty acids. It only makes sense that seafood has been the focus of health-related research because of its omega-3s.[6]

Eating more seafood is one way to, if I may say so, eat your way to better health. Most varieties of seafood are naturally low in sodium, fat, and calories while rich in protein and other nutrients. Seafood is generally a good source of the easily absorbed heme iron and contains B vitamins, vitamin D, potassium, magnesium, selenium, phosphorus, fluorine, sulfur, calcium, copper, and zinc.

Eating seafood supports bone health by providing both vitamin D and calcium. Sockeye salmon, mackerel, and tuna are excellent sources of vitamin D. Just a three ounce serving of canned sardines, bones included, provides more than a whopping 25% of the Dietary Reference Intake (DRI) for calcium. Even with the recent increase in the DRI for both vitamin D and calcium for adults ages 19 and over these two facts still hold true.[6]

Rank Your Catch of the Day

There is no dietary recommendation for omega-3 fatty acid intake. The DGA 2010, NHLBI, and American Heart Association recommend eating fish rich in omega-3 twice weekly for a total of about 8 to 12 ounces per week to enjoy its overall health benefits. Table 5.2 can help you see how your favorite seafood ranks nutritionally.

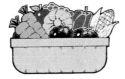

Table 5.2 Selected Seafood and Related Energy and Nutrient Contents

Species (3 oz., cooked)	Cal.	Fat (g)	Sat. fat (g)	Chol. (mg)	Omega-3 (g)
Mackerel, atlantic	223	15.1	3.6	64	1.2
Salmon, atlantic	155	6.9	1.1	60	2.2
Salmon, sockeye, bone included, canned	141	6.2	1.3	37	1.4
Herring, atlantic	173	9.9	2.2	65	1.9
Tuna, bluefin	156	5.3	1.4	42	1.4
Tuna, white, canned	109	2.5	0.7	36	0.8
Tuna, yellowfin	110	0.5	0.2	40	0.1
Halibut, atlantic	94	1.4	0.3	51	0.2
Bass, stripped	105	2.5	0.6	88	0.8
Trout, rainbow, wild	128	5.0	1.4	59	1.0
Trout, rainbow, farmed	143	6.3	1.4	60	0.9
Catfish	122	6.1	1.4	56	0.2
Snapper	109	1.5	0.3	40	0.3
Swordfish	146	6.7	1.6	66	0.9
Lobster	76	0.7	0.2	124	0.2
Crab, Alaska king	82	1.3	0.1	45	0.4
Crab, Alaska king, imitation, from surimi	81	0.4	0.2	17	<0.1
Shrimp, canned	85	1.2	0.2	214	0.5
Mollusks, scallop	94	0.7	0.2	35	0.2

Source: USDA National Nutrient Database for Standard Reference, Reference 23 (2010). Available at: http://www.ars.usda.gov/Services/docs.htm?docid=8964. Published October 2010. Accessed October 17, 2010.

Mercury and Seafood

Fish and shellfish are excellent sources of essential nutrients and healthy fats. They contribute to a balanced diet, healthy heart, and optimal growth and development of children. However, according to the FDA and the Environmental Protection Agency (EPA), nearly all fish and shellfish naturally contain traces of methyl mercury. According to both of these regulatory agencies, the trace amount isn't a health concern for most people. However, pregnant women and young children should limit consumption of fish high in methyl mercury as they can contribute to developmental problems, kidney, and irreversible nerve damage in the developing fetus.[7]

* * *

METHYL MERCURY: *What is mercury and methyl mercury? Mercury occurs naturally in the environment and can also be released into the air through industrial pollution. Mercury falls from the air near industrial sources and can accumulate in streams and oceans and turns into methyl mercury in the water. Fish absorb the methyl mercury as they feed in these waters and the chemical accumulates in the fish. Methyl mercury builds up considerably more in some types of fish and shellfish than others, depending on what the fish eat. It is this type of mercury that can be harmful to the unborn baby and young child.[7]*

* * *

Women who may become pregnant, those who are pregnant, nursing mothers, and young children should avoid some types of fish and eat only fish and shellfish that have lower mercury contents. According to the FDA and EPA these populations should follow three guidelines:

1. Avoid the four types of fish with the *highest* mercury content including king mackerel, shark, swordfish, and tilefish. Why these four? Because these larger fish have long life spans, allowing time for methyl mercury to accumulate in their bodies.

2. For women who are pregnant, plan to become pregnant, or who are breastfeeding, consume up to 12 ounces (two average meals) per week of a variety of fish and shellfish that are *lower* in mercury.

   • Five commonly eaten fish with *low* mercury content include shrimp, salmon, Pollock, catfish, and canned light tuna.

   • Albacore, also referred to as white, tuna has about twice the amount of mercury as canned light tuna. When choosing fish and shellfish as part of a meal choose up to six ounces (one average meal) of this type tuna per week.

3. Check local advisories regarding the safety of fish caught by relatives and friends who fish lakes, rivers, and coastal areas. If no advice is available, consume only six ounces per week of this type of fish and shellfish.[7]

When feeding children, use these same rules but serve smaller portions, generally two to three ounce instead of six ounce portions. This information about methyl mercury is rightfully alarming. However, it isn't necessary to stop eating all fish and be denied the benefits of its omega-3 containing benefits.[7]

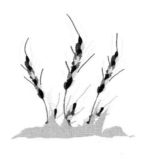

SIX

POWERFUL PRODUCE

All hail produce. All hail the mighty powers of vegetables and fruits. These are the only two food groups all RDs will agree should be on the all-you-can-eat menu. No one ever came to me overweight because they ate too much produce. These foods are the key to maintaining a healthy diet and are mighty disease fighters.

Health Benefits

Now it's time to embrace other members of the carbohydrate family, vegetables and fruits. Together vegetables and fruits supply vitamins, minerals, and fiber that collectively play an important role in reducing the risk of many chronic diseases. Vegetables and fruits are termed produce and important for good health. Eating a diet rich in produce:

- May reduce the risk for stroke and other cardiovascular diseases.
- May reduce the risk of type 2 diabetes.
- Protects against certain cancers, such as mouth, stomach, and colon-rectal cancer.

- May, because of their rich fiber content, reduce the risk of coronary heart disease by reducing blood cholesterol levels.

- May, because produce is rich in the mineral potassium, reduce the risk of developing kidney stones, may help to decrease bone loss, and may help maintain healthy blood pressure.

- Is naturally lower in calories, yet provides more volume, than other higher-calorie foods making produce useful in preventing obesity.[1,2]

A diet rich in produce begins with learning more about the vegetable and fruit groups.

The DGA 2010 confirmed that Americans consume insufficient amounts of folate, magnesium, potassium, dietary fiber and vitamins A, C, and K. This goes in step with its findings that Americans are poor consumers of produce. Of particular public health concern is the inadequate intake of potassium and dietary fiber necessary to support optimal health.[3] Having just discussed dietary fiber in Chapter 3 let's give some space to potassium going forward.

Vital Vegetables

Vegetables are the edible plant or plant parts whose definition or grouping is based more on culinary and cultural tradition. Some foods are thought to be vegetables, such as mushrooms or tomatoes, but they are actually fungi and fruit respectively. Most vegetables are low in calories and fat and never contain cholesterol. Nutritionally powerful, vegetables contain potassium, magnesium, folate, vitamin A in the form of beta-carotene, vitamin C, vitamin K, vitamin E, and dietary fiber.[1]

Vegetables rich in potassium include white beans, lima beans, kidney beans, beet greens, lentils, split peas, sweet potatoes, white potatoes, soybeans, spinach, winter squash, and tomato products.[1]

Of the vegetables rich in potassium, potatoes, beans, lentils, peas, soybeans, and winter squash are members of the starchy vegetable family. They are rich in vitamins and minerals, but also can contribute significant amounts of carbohydrate to the diet if eaten in unlimited amounts or prepared with fat, such as French fries. Starchy vegetables are considered to be part of a healthy diet and should not be avoided, but eaten in moderation.

Mighty Fruit

Fruits are naturally rich in carbohydrate, low in calories, sodium, and fat, and do not contain cholesterol. Nutritionally powerful, fruits contain dietary fiber and these nutrients: potassium, magnesium, folate, beta-carotene (vitamin A), and vitamin C. Fruits rich in potassium include bananas, prunes (dried plums), fresh and dried apricots, cantaloupe, honeydew melon, and prunes and orange juice.[2]

Daily Needs—Serving Sizes

Strive to eat 5 to 9 servings of produce daily. This can be easily achieved by choosing a variety of vegetables and fruits. For fruit specifically, select mostly whole and cut fruits rather than juice to benefit from its dietary fiber. Unless the juice is fortified with fiber it contains minimal amounts. Based on your gender, age, and activity level the specific amount of fruit to eat differs.

Depending on whether the vegetable or fruit is raw, cooked, dried, canned or frozen the serving size varies. Each of the following counts as one serving:

- 1 cup raw or ½ cup cooked vegetables
- 1 cup raw, leafy vegetables

- 1 medium-sized piece of fresh fruit or about four ounces

- 1/2 cup raw, cooked, frozen or canned fruits (in 100% juice)

- 1/2 of a grapefruit, papaya or mango

- 3/4 cup (6 ounces) 100% fruit or vegetable juice

- 1/2 cup cooked, canned or frozen legumes (beans and peas)

- 1/4 cup dried fruit[4,5]

Eat More Produce Tips

The ChooseMyPlate.gov website offers these and many more tips to encourage Americans to eat more produce daily:

- Plan some meals around a vegetable main dish, such as a vegetable stir-fry or soup. Then add other foods to complement it.

- Try a main dish salad for lunch. Go light on the salad dressing.

- Include a green salad with your dinner every night.

- Shred carrots or zucchini into meatloaf, casseroles, quick breads, and muffins.

- Include chopped vegetables in pasta sauce or lasagna.

- Order a veggie pizza with toppings like mushrooms, green peppers, and onions, and ask for extra veggies.

- Use pureed, cooked vegetables such as potatoes to thicken stews, soups and gravies. These add flavor, nutrients, and texture.

- Grill vegetable kebobs as part of a barbecue meal. Try tomatoes, mushrooms, green peppers, and onions.

- At breakfast, top your cereal with bananas or peaches; add blueberries to pancakes; drink 100% orange or grapefruit juice. Or, try a fruit mixed with low-fat or fat-free yogurt.

- At lunch, pack a tangerine, banana, or grapes to eat, or choose fruits from a salad bar. Individual containers of fruits like peaches or applesauce are easy and convenient.

- At dinner, add crushed pineapple to coleslaw, or include mandarin oranges or grapes in a tossed salad.

- Try meat dishes that incorporate fruit, such as chicken with apricots or mango chutney.

- Add fruit like pineapple or peaches to kabobs as part of a barbecue meal.

- For dessert, have baked apples, pears, or a fruit salad.[6,7]

Phytonutrients

Produce comes in a rainbow of colors with each tasty gem naturally containing *phytochemicals,* also known as *phytonutrients.* In Greek the word *phyto* means plant. These aren't the chemicals like those you have to keep out of the reach of children or read the warning label before using. Some foods which are excellent sources of phytochemicals may also be referred to as *functional foods* or foods that are not only nutritious, but may aid in specific body function in addition to reducing the risk of cancer and or heart disease. The term functional food was first introduced in Japan in the mid-1980s and refers to processed foods containing ingredients that aid specific bodily functions in addition to being nutritious. These are found in a tall glass of thirst quenching iced tea on a hot, summer day; a plump, juicy tomato just plucked from the vine, or in your morning bowl of oatmeal. For a review on functional foods see Chapter 2. Phytochemicals in food are a good thing.

Research has only begun to nail down the thousands or perhaps hundreds of thousands present in nature and the health benefit(s) of each one. Some phytonutrients, plant nutrients, serve the body by functioning as antioxidants to:

- patch up cells naturally damaged by cellular metabolism.

- protect cells from the effects of oxidation and free radicals in the body.

- potentially offer protection from diseases and conditions ranging from heart disease, and some cancers to aging.[8]

Since the early 1970s, researchers worldwide have reported that people who choose a primarily plant-based diet have lower rates of some types of cancers, a reduced risk of heart disease, osteoporosis, and less accelerated nerve cell damage. These observations have led to studies on the relationship of produce to decreased rates of disease.[9] Since the 1990s, the Nutrition Education and Labeling Act has regulated specific nutrition labeling on those foods claiming to have a disease or health related claim. These claims must be backed up by scientific evidence that the food or nutrient may prove beneficial as part of a healthy diet.

❋ ❋ ❋

ORANGE YOU HAPPY: *According to a study done in Australia, a single orange contains more than 170 different kinds of phytonutrients, each working to protect against unwanted intruders in your body.[10]*

❋ ❋ ❋

Think of phytochemicals as a *family tree* where each one is related to the other working in harmony to bring balance and health to the body. So far research has determined there are perhaps at least five main branches, families or classes of phytochemicals: alkaloids, carotenoids, organosulfurs, phenols and phytosterols.[11] Databases are limited on the phytochemical content of foods because the research on this topic is relatively new and a limited number of foods have been evaluated for their phytonutrient content.

Bear with me while I give you a taste for the vastness of the phytonutrient topic. Here is a glimpse into one phytonutrient family, the *phenols*. The phenol family has three major members or groups including flavonoids, stibenes, phenolic acids, and perhaps more. As a group, *flavonoids* contain at least six subgroups including isoflavones, anthocyanins, flavanones, flavones, flavonols and flavanols.[11]

Flavonoids are widely dispersed in the plant kingdom and are found in fruits, vegetables, tea, nuts, and seeds. Research has associated the consumption of foods containing flavonoids with a reduced risk of some chronic diseases.[11] Generally, flavonoids may help decrease the risk for certain types of cancer, boost the body's ability to defend against the damage to cells by free radicals, and promote both brain and heart health.[11-13]

The flavonoids, *isoflavones* (or phytoestrogens) are found in soybeans and soy-based foods (e.g., tofu, miso, and soybeans) and may help maintain healthy immune function, decrease the symptoms of menopause like hot flashes, reduce the risk of prostate and breast cancers, and support bone health following menopause.[12]

Another member of the flavonoid family is the *proanthocyanidins* that may help maintain both urinary tract and heart health. These are found in cranberries, grapes, cocoa, apples, strawberries, tea, and wine.[13,14] Grape juice, red grapes, red wine, peanuts and pistachios contain the phytonutrient *resveratrol*.[11] Resveratrol, found in the skin of red grapes and in red wine, may support heart health and reduce the risk of cardiovascular heart disease, stroke, blood clots, and cancer.[11,12]

● ● ●

DUI-GJ: *To consume red wine solely on its phytonutrient merits one should remember to do so in moderation, if at all, because it contains alcohol. Grape juice has a stronger nutrient profile than wine—read as vitamins, minerals, and contains no alcohol. Plus you can drink and drive while under the influence of grape juice! DUI-GJ.*

● ● ●

Sorting Benefits by Color

Most vegetables and fruits contain phytonutrients that contribute to taste, smell, and eye appeal. Phytonutrients can be sorted by color and produce type based on their natural plant pigments or colors. Here are some examples along with the health benefit each color offers.

Green

This produce group color comes from the plant pigment *chlorophyll*. Some members of this group also contain lutein, a powerful cartenoid that may help keep eyes healthy and protect against macular degeneration and cataracts. Indoles found in cabbage, broccoli sprouts and cauliflower may help protect again certain types of cancer.[15,16]

Examples include avocados, green grapes, kiwifruit, green peas, green apples, honeydew, artichokes, asparagus, broccoli sprouts, broccoli, green beans, green peppers, and leafy greens.[15]

Red

Plant pigments called *lycopene* or *anthocyanins* contribute to the red shades of this group. Lycopene, a potent cartenoid, found in watermelon, tomatoes and pink grapefruit may decrease the risk of certain types of cancer, particularly prostate cancer.[13,15] The anthocyanins found in red grapes and strawberries may help promote healthy vision, promote heart health, and boost immunity.[15,16]

Examples include watermelon, red/pink grapefruit, raspberries, cherries, cranberries, pomegranates, red grapes, tomatoes, beets, red peppers, red onions, and rhubarb.[15]

Yellow/Orange

This produce group is colored by the plant pigments called carotenoids. Beta-carotene is the primary carotenoid that is converted by the body into vitamin A which is known to promote healthy skin and night vision. The carotenoids and the powerful antioxidant vitamin C found in this group may help promote heart health, immunity, and may reduce the risk of some cancers.[13,15]

Examples include mangos, peaches, papayas, cantaloupe, apricots, peaches, butternut squash, carrots, yellow peppers, pumpkin, yellow corn, and sweet potatoes.[15]

Blue/Purple

The purple-blue plant pigments called *anthocyanins* help give plants their deep purples, blues, and dark reds color. The skins of red grapes contain this pigment. Anthocyanins found in blueberries, raisins, and black grapes act as potent antioxidants that may protect cells from damage, and may reduce the risk of heart disease, stroke and some types of cancer.[15,16] Some studies link the ample intake of the anthocyanins found in blueberries to healthy aging and helping memory function.[15]

Examples include mulberries, blackberries, plums, raisins, purple, grapes, blueberries, figs, eggplant, and purple-fleshed potatoes.[15]

White/Tan/Brown

This group is colored by plant pigments called *anthoxanthins*.[15] Onions, garlic, leeks and scallions from the allium class of bulb shaped plants called *allium* contain the phytonutrients *allyl sulfides*. These phytonutrients may function as a detoxifier for the body, support heart health, and a healthy immune system.[12,13] Specifically the phytonutrient, *allicin* found in onions and garlic may help lower blood pressure, cholesterol, and lower the risk of stomach cancer.[15]

Examples include bananas, white peaches, white nectarines, brown pears, dates, cauliflower, white cabbage, garlic, jicama, kohlrabi, onions, mushrooms, onions, white corn, turnips, and white potatoes.[15]

* * *

THE SAILOR GOT HER C: *I recently travelled with a group of medical providers to South Korea in support of a military training exercise. Once the two-week training was complete we were awarded several hours of time off (liberty) to relax, venture out and mingle with the locals. Ann, a fellow military dietitian and vegetarian, asked me to accompany her in a visit to a South Korean family's home in the area where we were staying. During the visit I experienced fresh kiwi and baked sweet potatoes in the purest of forms. The plump kiwis, in season at the time, were cut into fourths and served skin and all. The skin is rich in fiber.[17] The sweet potatoes (naturally containing iron) had been washed and baked in their skins and served with the skin on like a whole banana. The natural sweetness of both was fantastic. Kiwi and sweet potatoes are packed with phytonutrients and vitamin C.[14] Different cultures can teach us about what they consider tasty, special and nutritious about food.*

* * *

Nutrition in a Nutshell

Nuts, besides being a rich source of monounsaturated and polyunsaturated fats, also contain phytonutrients and are super foods created in nature. Nomadic people first gathered nuts growing in the wild. Around 10,000 BC people began to cultivate and farm nut trees. Most nuts are the dried fruit or seeds of trees. Most have hard, woody outer husks that protect its soft inner seed or kernel.[18]

Nuts are very powerful sources of energy and a few go a long way. Nuts contain little to no water and are generally high in fat and thus, calories. In addition to being a good source of plant-based protein, nuts are also a source of vitamins, minerals, heart healthy fats, and a dab of carbohydrate. Because nuts come from plants and plants don't have a heartbeat (except in the cartoons) they are cholesterol-free. One ounce (about a handful) of pistachios, pine nuts, or hazelnuts has about 165 calories.[19]

Between 8% to 18% of a nut's calories are from protein. Lacking the essential amino acid, lysine, nuts are considered an incomplete protein source. Nuts have the potential to serve the same function to the body as an animal-based protein if it joins the amino acid lysine from another food source to make it complete.

Nuts are one of the best plant sources of vitamin E which is found in its oil-rich kernels. Nuts are a source of B vitamins thiamin, niacin, and riboflavin. Potassium and iron are found in almonds, Brazil nuts, and filberts. The filbert is a good source of calcium. Nuts also contain the minerals magnesium, copper and selenium in varying amounts.[19]

● ● ●

BLACK WALNUT FACTS: *The product of a tree native to North America, the black walnut is a tasty nut enjoyed by many. The black walnut drops from its tree surrounded by an outer green husk where it ripens before it is released to the elements to dry. It is a finely tuned product of nature. The black walnut has* *a dark, very hard shell that requires significant pressure to crack open. The black walnut, like the Persian (or English) walnut, is a healthy source of calories, protein, cholesterol-free fat, and negligible fiber. Black walnuts contain 175 calories, 1.9 grams of dietary fiber, 6.8 grams of protein and 16.7 grams of fat per one-eighth cup serving.[19]*

● ● ●

Tea—Drink and Thrive

Ah! Tea...it quenches your thirst on a sizzling summer day and is as cozy and satisfying as a warm pair of socks in the winter. Tea has been served as a beverage for centuries, and it remains one of the world's most popular drinks, second only to water. Tea is both inexpensive and one of the simplest beverages to prepare. One pound of tea will yield about 200 cups, compared to a pound of coffee which yields about 40 cups.

Tea naturally contains ingredients, including phytonutrients, which help the body fight disease by protecting healthy cells and tissues against damage. Researchers continue to examine the role tea plays in fighting cancer and heart disease. Tea may help reduce the risk of some forms of cancer and help reduce blood cholesterol levels.[20,21]

Tea is a Species of the Evergreen Shrub, You Say?

How many kinds of tea are there? One. The name of the plant from which all teas are produced is *Camellia sinensis*, a species of the evergreen shrub. The three main categories of tea are derived from how each one is processed. Names of the subcategories are then labeled according to where the tea was grown geographically.

The three categories of tea include black, green and oolong. There are more than 3,000 different varieties of teas based on where they are grown and how they are fermented or processed. The fermentation process takes place by the action of enzymes naturally occurring in the tea leaves.

- Black tea is most popular in the United States, Great Britain, Europe, and India. It is fermented by exposing the newly harvested leaves to air in a damp place. This natural chemical process is what produces its deep red-brown color and unique rich flavor. The term Orange Pekoe refers to the specific leaf size of any black variety of tea and is not a variety of tea itself. Some varieties of black tea include: Assam, Ceylon, Darjeeling, Earl Grey, English Breakfast, Keemun, and Souchong.

- Green tea is my favorite and popular in Japan, China and becoming a favorite in the United States. It is dried without fermenting. Green tea is naturally processed by quick steaming or heating of the raw tea leaves. Jasmine and chrysanthemum teas are a blend of dry flowers combined with either green or black tea. Some other green tea varieties include: Sencha, Gunpower, and Jasmine.

- Oolong tea is probably the most popular tea in China. It is semi-fermented and is a combination of both green and black tea. It has a greenish-brown color. The taste of good quality oolong tea is peachy and mellow. Some varieties include: Formosa, Oolong Orange Blossom, Orchid Oolong and Ti Kuan Yin Iron Goddess tea.[20-24]

Herbal Tisanes

Noteworthy is the topic of herbal teas, or more appropriately termed, *tisanes*. Tisanes don't come from the *Camellia sinensis* plant and aren't really teas. Tisanes are a collection of plant leaves, herbs, spices, roots, flowers and flavorings steeped in hot water to make an infusion. Some varieties of tisanes include: Chamomile, Lemon Rose and Peppermint. This section refers to teas from *Camellia sinensis* only.[20-22,24] Sometimes tisanes are added to teas to add variety and flavor.

The Drink for Good Health

Enjoyed by civilizations for at least 5,000 years, tea was first identified by Chinese scholars for its medicinal attributes. Today, scientists continue to study tea's potential role in the prevention of heart disease and cancer. The results of current research are positive, exciting and have made tea even more popular.[20,21,24]

Tea, like fruits, vegetables, nuts and seeds, contains a variety of phytochemicals. The antioxidants in tea may help to keep body cells and tissues healthy and slow down the aging process. Antioxidants in tea are thought to be effective in preventing heart disease by promoting mild reductions in serum low-density lipoproteins (LDL) while restoring blood vessel dilation to near normal levels in persons with heart disease.[20,21,25]

Polyphenols, powerful antioxidants, are naturally occurring chemical components of tea. Some researchers have determined that drinking tea may decrease your chances of getting cavities by suppressing the growth of cavity-causing bacteria in dental plaque and reducing acid production. Dental plaque causes gum disease, a leading cause of tooth loss in adults.[20,21,26]

In addition, polyphenols found in green tea have been found to be an inhibitor of some types of cancer and various other diseases. Dry tea has been said to exceed the antioxidant activity of more than 22 vegetables and fruit, and the benefits range from reducing the risk of oral, digestive, and colon cancers to stroke. Research continues on the risks and benefits of tea consumption. Additional scientific studies on the role of the antioxidants in tea must be done to make conclusions regarding its contributions to health.[20,21,25,26]

One consequence yet to be fully explored is the possibility of a drug-food interaction when green teas are consumed with certain drugs.[20,21] Examples include those used to treat depression like monoamine oxidase inhibitors (MAOIs) and anticoagulants like Warfarin.

Tea and Caffeine

Tea naturally contains about one-half the amount of caffeine per cup as coffee. What's a safe amount of caffeine to consume on a daily basis? Most healthy adults can drink about two to three cups of medium brewed coffee, or 200 to 300 mg of caffeine per day. Translated into tea-terms, that is equivalent to about five cups of medium brewed tea. The longer the tea steeps, the higher the caffeine content in the tea. Go with the decaffeinated variety of your favorite of tea if caffeine is causing you insomnia, irritability or stomach distress. For health benefits, one to four cups of tea per day have been shown to be beneficial for cardiovascular disease reduction.[20,21,24] If you drink large amounts of tea be sure to read any drug inserts and to ask your nutrition professional, physician or pharmacist about any potential adverse effects. Switching to decaffeinated beverages may be all that is necessary for you to enjoy your tea and reap its health benefits. Remember to take prescription medications as directed.

Tea Made Right

For a good cup of traditional tea, follow these directions and you'll be a success:

1. One teaspoon of loose tea or one single serve tea bag will make a bright 6-oz cup of tea.

2. Rinse the cup or teapot with hot water to warm up the container. Always use a china, stainless steel or glass container. Other metals may give off a flavor.

3. Bring cold, fresh water to a boil (212°F). Warm water will make flat-tasting tea.

4. Place the tea bag or the loose tea leaves in the pot and pour the water directly over the leaves.

5. Allow the tea to steep (let stand to extract flavors and colors) 3 to 5 minutes.

6. Serve immediately as tea doesn't hold well.[20,21,27]

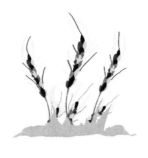

SEVEN

FOOD AFTER 50

The Serenity Prayer: God, give us grace to accept with serenity the things that cannot be changed, courage to change the things which should be changed, and the wisdom to distinguish the one from the other.
—Reinhold Niebuhr (1892-1971)

Time Travel—The Fabulous 50s and Beyond

Chronological age means little compared to your attitude and outlook on life and health. Applying your knowledge, experience, and wisdom to what life tosses your way day-by-day can make traveling through time a beautiful thing. Tweaking eating habits to match energy needs and activity levels is a smart way to maintain a healthy body weight and stay healthy. You are what you eat. Strive to be a carrot body instead of a muffin body.

Guides to Eat By

If your past eating habits included the basic *see-food diet*—you see the food and you eat it, it may be time for a change. The USDA and the Department of Health and Human Service (DHHS) offer two eating plans or patterns to get the nutrients to maintain good health. The first is the USDA Food Patterns and its vegetarian variation. As we age muscle mass tends to decrease and fat accounts for more of your weight, slowing down calorie burning. Metabolism is also thought to slow down as we age contributing to the need for fewer calories as well.

The USDA MyPlate Food Patterns (replacing MyPyramid) suggests that people age 51 and beyond eat a balanced diet with nutritious choices from the following food groups each day:

- Fruits: 1½ to 2 cups
  What is the same as 1/2 cup of cut-up fruit? *One medium whole fruit or ¼ cup of dried fruit.*

- Vegetables: 2 to 2½ cups
  What is the same as a cup of cut-up vegetables? *Two cups of uncooked leafy vegetables.*

- Grains: 5 to 6 ounces
  What is the same as an ounce of grains? *One roll, a small muffin, a slice of bread, 1 cup of flaked, ready-to-eat cereal, or ½ cup of cooked rice, pasta, or cereal.*

- Protein Foods: 5 to 5½ ounces equivalents
  What is the same as an ounce of meat, fish, or poultry? *One egg, ¼ cup of cooked beans or tofu, ½ ounce of nuts or seeds, or 1 tablespoon of peanut butter.*

- Dairy: 3 cups of fat-free or low-fat milk
  What is the same as 1 cup of milk? *One cup of yogurt or 1-1/2 to 2 ounces of cheese. One cup of cottage cheese is the same as ½ cup of milk.*[1]

Notice the eating plan does not indicate a need for special foods, fat substitutes or supplements. Depending on your current health, your medical provider may recommend that you follow a special diet that includes or restricts certain foods. Health problems like diabetes, heart disease or hypertension may improve with diet therapy. Some medications work better when certain foods are restricted in your diet. Ask your provider or a registered dietitian about what foods you can eat instead to replace those foods restricted. Remember always opt to get the nutrients you need through the foods you eat rather than a potion or pill.[2]

DASH for Good Health

The second eating plan is the *Dietary Approach to Stop Hypertension Eating Plan or DASH*. The DGA 2010 recommend adopting healthy eating habits by implementing the USDA Food Patterns or the NHLBI DASH eating plan.[3] The DASH eating plan is a component of the NHLBI's TLC program to help reduce and prevent heart disease as discussed in Chapter 5 which also calls for increased physical activity, decreased alcohol consumption and stopping smoking. This eating plan provides dietary guidance originally developed to help lower blood pressure that is flexible and is easy to follow regardless of your current health. The DASH eating plan focuses on eating foods already easily available from your grocer, farmer's market, or garden. It focuses on eating:

- More vegetables and fruits.

- More fat-free or low-fat milk and milk products.

- More whole grains.

- Foods low in saturated fat, cholesterol and total fat.

- Fish, poultry, beans, seeds and nuts.

- Fewer sweets, added sugars and sugary drinks, and red meats than the typical American diet.

- Less sodium and salt than the typical American diet.[4]

Notice that DASH does not indicate a need for special foods, fat substitutes or supplements. The USDA Food Patterns and its vegetarian variation work nicely as a guide for putting DASH into action. The *resource section* in the *general health resources and disease prevention section* provides more detailed information on the DASH eating plan plus a link to the NHLBI website. I recommend using one or both of the plans for healthy eating. Eating a variety of foods from each food group in either plan will help you get the nutrients you need.

Regardless of which one you choose it's always a good idea to shy away from empty calories from food and beverages heavy in calories but light in nutrients such as chips, cookies, sodas, and alcohol.[2]

The Balancing Act

Eating the smaller recommended amounts from each food group in the USDA Food Patterns equals about 1600 calories. Eating the larger amounts from each food group equals about 2800 calories. Remember that calories are a way to count how much energy a food contains. Energy you get from the food you eat helps you do the things you need to do each day—plus those you do to have fun!

If you've traveled past age 50 use Table 7.1 as a general guide to determine your daily calorie level.

Table 7.1 Calories Consumed Matched To Calories Used

ACTIVITY LEVEL	FEMALE*	MALE*
Not physically active	1600	2000
Somewhat active	1800	2200-2400
Active lifestyle	2000-2200	2400-2800

*Healthy adults 50 years of age and over
Source: National Institute on Aging. Eating healthy after 50. Available at: http://www.nia.nih.
gov/healthinformation/publications/healthyeating.htm. Updated October 5, 2010. Accessed Oct
28, 2010.

Just counting calories is not enough for making healthy food choices. For example, a medium banana, 1 cup of unsweetened flaked cereal, 2 ½ cups of cooked spinach, 1 tablespoon of peanut butter, or 1 cup of 1% milk all have roughly the same number of calories. But, the foods are different in many ways. Some have more of the nutrients you might need than others. Milk gives you more calcium than a banana, and peanut butter gives you more protein than cereal. And a banana is likely to make you feel full more than a tablespoon of peanut butter.[2] Choose wisely.

Let your activity level drive the amount you eat. If you take in more calories than you expend you may gain weight. The opposite is true for expending more calories than you consume where you may lose weight. Strive to match your activity level with the amount of calories you eat. Along with eating healthy, the more active you are the more likely you will prevent, delay or lessen the onset of health problems. Do your best to get 30 minutes of moderate activity every day.[2]

* * *

DO NEEDS CHANGE?: *Yes and no. Nutrient needs including protein, calcium, vitamin A, vitamin C, vitamin D, vitamin B12, iron, folic acid, zinc and water remain the same as in your younger years but the amounts change. You can help prevent osteoporosis, high blood pressure, obesity, diabetes, heart disease, stroke and some types of cancer by eating a healthy diet. Eat a diet rich in produce, dietary fiber, plant-based proteins, low-fat dairy, whole*

grains with moderate consumption of lean meat and minimum
amounts of saturated fat, salty foods, and alcohol, if at all.[5]

● ● ●

Serving Right-Sizing

How does the food on your plate compare to recommended portion sizes? For example, one very large chicken breast could be more from the protein foods group than is recommended for a whole day. Here are some general ways you can check:

- 3 ounces of meat, poultry, or fish = a deck of card

- ½ cup of fruit, rice, pasta, or ice cream = ½ baseball

- 1 cup of salad greens = a baseball

- 1 teaspoon of butter or margarine = a dice (or die)

- 2 tablespoons of peanut butter = a ping pong ball

- 1 cup of flaked cereal or a baked potato = a small fist[2]

Read the Label

At first, reading labels on many packaged foods may take some time. The Nutrition Facts panel found on all boxed, bagged, processed, and some fresh foods, tells how much protein, carbohydrates, fats, sodium, key vitamins and minerals, and calories are in a serving. The panel also shows how many servings are in the package—be careful because sometimes what you think is one serving is really more. Each can, bottle, or package label also has an ingredients list. Items are listed from largest amount to smallest.[2] Turn to Appendix A for details on label reading.

Fiber Focus

Of particular importance as you age is to eat adequate amounts of dietary fiber for good digestion, regular elimination, and optimal bowel function. Getting adequate fiber can naturally help prevent constipation and other stomach and bowel problems. Constipation is more related to how well you're eating and how much water you're drinking than your age. We learned in Chapter 3 about fiber sources and quantities to consume based on our age. Use those guidelines and remember it's always better to get fiber from foods instead of dietary supplements.

Should You Shake the Salt?

The most common source of sodium, a part of salt, is from processed foods. Those foods that are boxed, bagged, or packaged usually come with a hefty helping of sodium. Most people when told to reduce their sodium intake, state, "I do not use the salt shaker" or "I don't put salt on my food." Adding salt from the shaker to food is no longer the main source of sodium in the American diet. The body needs sodium, but too much can make blood pressure go up in some people. Most fresh food contains some sodium naturally. Salt is added to many canned and prepared foods to enhance flavor or act as a preservative.[2]

People tend to eat more salt than they need. If you are over age 50, 1500 mg of sodium or about 2/3 teaspoon of salt (table or sea salt) is all you need each day. That is not just from the salt shaker but also includes sodium in your food and drink. If your doctor tells you to use less salt, ask about a salt substitute. Some contain sodium and some may contain potassium that can interfere with certain medication. Avoid adding salt during cooking or at the table, and avoid salty snacks and processed foods. Look for the word sodium, not just the word salt, on the Nutrition

Facts panel. Choose foods labeled low-sodium. Often, the amount of sodium in the same kind of food can vary greatly between brands.[2]

⬤　⬤　⬤

A FLAVOR TIP: *Spices, herbs, vinegars and lemon juice can add flavor to your food, so you won't miss the salt.*

⬤　⬤　⬤

Fluid Focus

Fiber needs ample amounts of fluids to move through your gut and be eliminated. Water is the only nutrient you can't get enough of from food alone. With age sometimes comes a diminished sense of thirst. In Chapter 2 you learned that drinking enough fluid daily including water, milk, juice, and soup can help you stay hydrated. Remind yourself to drink plenty of liquids daily even when you aren't thirsty. Urine that is pale yellow indicates you are well hydrated. If your urine is dark or bright yellow you may need more fluids. Never stop drinking fluids to solve a bladder control problem. Trouble with controlling urine output is reason enough to consult your medical provider.[2]

Food Frustration

Does your favorite food not taste and smell the same as it used to? While these changes may be frustrating, neither is unusual. The sense of smell and sense of taste may diminish as you travel through time. Certain medicines can change or decrease your appetite and tastes. Ask your pharmacist and medical provider about alternative medications if the side effects are keeping you from eating a variety of foods. Add more herbs or spices to your foods to enhance their flavor.[2]

If you find that milk-containing foods you used to eat or drink without problems are now resulting in symptoms of gas, stomach pain or diarrhea you may be experiencing lactose intolerance. Don't try to guess if you are lactose intolerant or not as you may actually have another problem; ask your doctor to test you. Lactose intolerance happens when your body is missing the enzyme lactase, necessary to effectively breakdown the milk sugar lactose naturally found in dairy foods. Some individuals can eat limited amounts of dairy products without having symptoms while others can only tolerate buttermilk, yogurt or hard cheese. Luckily many lactose-free foods are available. Consult your medical provider to determine whether or not you're lactose intolerant. Adequate intake of calcium should be addressed if you're not able to eat dairy products.[2]

If you're unable to enjoy your favorite foods because it's harder to chew it's time to consult your dentist. Sore gums, loose teeth or poorly fitting dentures can cause pain and discomfort making eating mechanically difficult.[2] Eating softer and easier to chew foods are options until you can be examined by a dentist and get the problems remedied. Good oral hygiene is critical for the maximum enjoyment of food at any age. I love my dentist, Dr. Thomas, and I hope you find one you can love, too.

Move It—Move It—Move It ...OR LOSE IT

Regular physical activity is beneficial regardless of your age. Staying active may help you:

- Perk up your mood and reduce depression
- Keep and improve your strength so you can stay independent
- Stay flexible so you can do all the maneuvers you did at age 30

- Have more energy and endurance to do the things you want to do

- Improve your balance

- Prevent or delay some diseases like heart disease, diabetes, breast and colon cancer, and osteoporosis[6]

You don't need to buy special clothes or belong to a gym to become more active. Physical activity can and should be part of your everyday life. Find things you like to do and do them. Go for brisk walks, ride a bicycle or join a spin class, dance, do spring cleaning—often, garden, climb stairs whenever you can, swim or try water aerobics. The choices are limitless. Try different kinds of activities that keep you moving. Look for new ways to build physical activity into your daily routine.[6]

Local fitness centers or hospitals might be able to help you find a physical activity program that works for you. You could also ask your physician to refer you to a physical therapist if you have a bad back, sore joints, or have not exercised for months or years. You also can check with nearby houses of worship, senior and civic centers, parks and recreation associations, YMCAs, YWCAs, or even shopping malls for exercise, wellness, or walking programs.[6]

Looking for more information on how to exercise safely? The Exercise and Physical Activity: Your Everyday Guide from the National Institute on Aging (NIA) has strength, balance, and stretching exercises you can do at home. You can order this free guide from the NIA Information Center by mail or online. Many national organizations have information about physical activity and exercise for older adults.[6] See the *resource section* listed under *nutrition and aging.*

Always check with your doctor if you aren't used to lively, vigorous activity. Regardless your past level of activity, a regular check-up is a good idea at any age and especially when starting a new fitness routine. Regardless of your age remember to approach any activity starting slowly with a good warm-up and end with a cool-down after each workout. Enjoy!

Are You Lonely Tonight?

Aging can sometimes mean out-living your loved ones or out-loving some relationships. Here are some social solutions if you find yourself wanting company especially during mealtime:

- Cash in on the early bird specials when portions are smaller and prices are lower—that's when many people like you may be dining.

- Sit at the counter in your favorite diner—it's a great place to dine with other solo diners.

- Play your favorite music or radio program during mealtime to give you some company.

- Pack yourself a bag lunch and go eat in the park. The scenery is great and let nature provide the entertainment.

- Whip up some of your favorite homemade foods and place them in one to two portion containers and freeze for upcoming meals.

- Invite some friends over for a meal or plan a mini-buffet with each guest contributing food to the feast.

- Take the time to set the table with your best china and silver. After all, *who are you saving all that stuff for anyway!* Use it. Enjoy it. Be your own special guest. It will boost your spirits and may inspire a diminishing appetite.

- If you want a change of pace, try out the local Senior Center for lunch. You'll be amazed to see the reasonable prices and the great time folks are having. Make new friends and get reacquainted with old friends. The centers usually provide daily activities, excursions, dancing and various other social opportunities.[5] Among the activities often offered is Bingo, Mom's favorite sport.

Boost Immunity

As you are out and about getting acquainted and reacquainted with the world, plan on boosting your immune system before and during the flu and cold season. The more compromised your health the more vulnerable you are to the flu. Combine the factors of increased stress during a typical holiday season, mixed with unhealthy eating and decreased exercise and you have a recipe for catching the bug. In addition, both drinking enough fluids and nutrition play vital roles in reducing the risks for getting the flu while also fighting against chronic diseases like heart disease, diabetes, certain cancers and osteoporosis.

Join the Immunity Booster Club

As we learned in the section on phytonutrients, it's a fact that vitamins and minerals, from the foods we eat and drink, serve important roles in helping boost immunity. Fruits and vegetable are perhaps the most important of the food groups in flu prevention and for boosting the immune system. We know the body needs nutrients from all five food groups plus plenty of fluids for overall health maintenance. Probiotics, also called good bacteria or friendly bacteria, may have a beneficial effect by helping balance the microflora in the gut, improving gastrointestinal (GI) function and overall immunity. Prebiotics and probiotics found in or added to foods may result in improved GI tract function and better overall health. Refer to Chapter 2 for food sources of these functional foods.

The Center for Disease Control and Prevention (CDC) indicates the single most important prevention tool to keep from getting the flu is to get an annual flu shot. Second to getting a flu shot is to wash your hands regularly. Year round, putting these two tips into action can help keep you well.[7]

Additionally, the CDC suggests five more savvy ways to help prevent getting the flu. Note all of these tools are of equal importance.

- *Avoid close contact.* Avoid close contact with people who are sick. When you are sick, keep your distance from others to protect them from getting sick too.

- *Stay home when you are sick.* If possible, stay home from work, school, and errands when you are sick. You may help prevent others from catching your illness.

- *Cover your mouth and nose.* Cover your mouth and nose with a tissue when coughing or sneezing. It may help prevent those around you from getting sick.

- *Avoid touching your eyes, nose or mouth.* Germs are often spread when a person touches something that is contaminated with germs and then touches his or her eyes, nose, or mouth.

- *Practice other good health habits.* Get plenty of sleep, be physically active, manage your stress, drink plenty of fluids, and eat nutritious food.[7]

Keeping Food Safe

As you age and or if your immune system is compromised extra care must be taken to keep food safe to eat. As you get older, you are less able to fight off infections, and some foods could make you very sick or worse yet, kill you. Be sure to fully cook eggs, pork, fish, shellfish, poultry, and hot dogs. Talk to your doctor or a registered dietitian about foods to avoid. Some foods to avoid might include raw sprouts, some deli meats, and foods that are not pasteurized (heated to destroy disease-causing organisms) like some milk products and juices in the refrigerated section of the grocery.[2]

Before cooking, handle raw meat, poultry, or fish with care. Keep these raw items apart from foods that are already cooked or won't be cooked, like salad, fruit, or bread. Be careful with kitchen tools—your knife, plate, or cutting board, for example. Don't cut raw meat with the same knife you will use to make a salad without washing it with soap and water. Rinse raw fruits and vegetables before eating. Remember, the first defense against any illness is good hand hygiene. Use hot soapy water to wash your hands, tools, and work surfaces as you cook.[2]

As you get older, you can't depend on sniffing or tasting food to tell if it has gone bad. And many foods that have gone bad do not have an off odor or taste. Label and date foods stored in your refrigerator. Check the *use by* date on foods. If in doubt, toss it out.[2]

● ● ●

TO KEEP OR TOSS: *Refrigerate cooked food within 2 hours of it being cooked—whether it's home-cooked or from a restaurant.*

● ● ●

Thrifty Healthy Eating Options

If your budget is limited, it might take some thought and planning to be able to afford the foods you should eat. Here are some suggestions that might be helpful:

- First, buy only the foods you need. A shopping list will help with that.

- Before shopping, plan your meals, and check your supply of staples like flour and cereal.

- Make sure you have some canned or frozen foods in case you do not feel like cooking or cannot go out. Powdered, canned, or ultra-pasteurized milk in a shelf carton can be stored easily.

- Think about how much of a food you will use. A large size may be cheaper per unit, but it is only a bargain if you use all of it.

- Try to share large packages of food with a friend. Frozen vegetables in bags save money because you can use small amounts and keep the rest frozen. If a package of meat or fresh produce is too large, ask a store employee to repackage it in smaller sized packages.[2]

Here are other ways to keep food costs down:

- Plain (generic) labels or store brands often cost less than name brands.

- Plan your meals around food that is on sale.

- Prepare more of the foods you enjoy, and quickly refrigerate the leftovers to eat within a couple days.

- Divide leftovers into small servings, label and date, and freeze to use within a few months.[2]

Can't make your financial ends meet no matter how hard you try? The Supplemental Nutrition Assistance Program (SNAP) previously called the Food Stamp Program is a USDA funded program that's been in existence since the War on Poverty and helps people with low incomes buy healthy food. You may be able to enjoy free or low-cost meals for older people at a community center, church, or school. This is a chance to eat good food and to be with other people. Home-delivered meals are available for people who are homebound.[2] To learn more refer to the *resource section* under *nutrition and aging.*

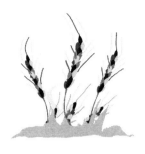

RIGHT SIZE YOUR FOOD, FIGURE AND FITNESS

The good feelings follow the action
—not the other way around.

—Howard Liebgold, M.D.

Size Matters

Regardless of your age, there is a relationship between what you eat, how much you eat, your body weight, your fitness level, and your overall health. These are all interdependent. In a quest for healthy living, it is important that you evaluate all five. Getting into action to eat right can result in better long term health. Action includes right sizing the portions of food you eat, right sizing your body weight to within a healthy range, and choosing your optimum activity level. You've learned what to eat in earlier chapters. Now it's time to learn about how much food enough is, what a healthy body weight is, and activity for overall healthy results.

Right Size Your Portion

It's vital to be completely honest with yourself when examining your eating habits. The scale doesn't lie nor do your clothes. What counts as a *portion* is often different from what counts as a *serving*. A portion is the amount of food you eat. You decide how big or small the amount is. A serving is a specific amount of food or drink established by the food manufacturer. That amount may or may not fit into USDA's idea of what a serving to meet your nutritional needs is. Nutrition recommendations are based on serving sizes of the basic food groups to help us understand the amounts we should eat of a variety of foods to get the nutrients we for good health. Sometimes we eat a portion that is equal to a serving, sometimes we eat more.[1]

If you eat a large portion of food make sure you know how many servings it is and count it as such. For example, a serving of pasta is one-third to one-half cup but a dinner portion of pasta is often as much as three to six servings. Although one serving, according to the food label, is two ounces or about one cup (at least twice the amount of a recommended serving), that one cup comes with about 45 grams of carbohydrate and up to 240 calories, so be careful when judging how much pasta you are eating. The same is true for rice and other starchy foods. Easy does it.

Like those examples introduced in Chapter 7, here are some more portion control guidelines and comparisons to help you decide whether your portion sizes are in control:

- One ounce of meat—a match box

- Three ounces of meat—a deck of cards or medium bar of soap

- Eight ounces of meat—a thin paperback book that could fit in your coat pocket

- A medium apple or orange—a tennis ball

- A medium potato—a computer mouse

- One cup of lettuce—four leaves of head lettuce
- One ounce of cheese—four dice
- One cup of fruit—a baseball or a small fist

Compare these portion sizes with those you normally eat. Cut back or add on if necessary. Implementing reasonable portion sizes can help you trim down a few pounds without much effort and vice versa. Listed below are the serving sizes for a portion of food from the five food groups plus oils and fats:

- Grains: 1 slice of bread, 1 ounce of ready-to-eat cereal, 1/2 cup of cooked cereal, rice, or pasta.

- Vegetables: 1 cup of raw leafy vegetables, 1/2 cup of other vegetables, cooked or chopped raw, 3/4 cup of vegetable juice. Potatoes, corn, lima beans are vegetables but are often called starchy vegetables because their calorie and carbohydrate content are much more than non-starchy vegetables such as broccoli, carrots, greens, and tomatoes.

- Fruits: 1 medium piece of fruit; 1/2 cup of chopped, cooked, or canned fruit; 3/4 cup of fruit juice.

- Protein Foods: 2-3 ounces of cooked lean meat, poultry, or fish; 1/2 cup of cooked dry beans, 1 egg; 1 tablespoon of peanut butter and 1 ounce of nuts count as 1 ounce of high fat meat.

- Dairy: 1 cup of milk or yogurt, 1 1/2 ounces of natural cheese, 2 ounces of processed cheese.

- Oils and Fats: 1 tablespoon vegetable oil, mayonnaise or mayonnaise-type salad dressing; 2 tablespoons salad dressing; 4 large, ripe olives; 1/2 medium avocado, 1 ounce nuts; 1 teaspoon butter or stick margarine.[2]

Mabel, Mabel Read the Label

Having a general understanding of the health and nutrient content claims on food labels is a must to make informed and healthy choices when you shop. Food labeling and the health claims on food packaging can add a significant amount of understanding or confusion to the shopper. Appendix A contains a general guide on how to read and understand the nutrition facts label on foods.

Millions of dollars are invested in food marketing to promote and market a product manufacturers and advertisers want to convince you that you just cannot live without. Being able to make positive health claims and nutrient content claims on a product label can make all the difference in the sale or fail of a product. Any single food label may contain many different kinds of claims. The FDA regulates all claims making sure the information presented is accurate and science based.

A *health claim* relates a disease or health condition to a nutrient or substance found in a food. The FDA allows these types of claims on food labels, as well as nutrient content claims if there is research to back them up. Examples include dietary fat and cancer; sodium and hypertension; grain products, vegetables and fruit containing fiber and cancer; calcium and osteoporosis; dietary saturated fat and cholesterol and coronary heart disease risk.[3,4,5] Here's an example of a health claim from a box of oatmeal, *"Three grams of soluble fiber from oatmeal every day, in a diet low in saturated fat and cholesterol, may reduce the risk of heart disease."*

Defining Nutrient Claims

A *nutrient content claim* defines how much of a nutrient there is in a food. Some examples of nutrient claims include:

- Free—contains none or a very small amount of the nutrient

- Calorie free—less than 5 calories per serving

- Fat free—less than 0.5 grams of fat per serving

- Sugar free—less than 0.5 grams of sugar per serving

- Low in—can be used on foods eaten often without exceeding the dietary guidelines for that specific nutrient

- Low calorie—less than 40 calories per serving

- Low fat—3 grams or less per serving

- Low cholesterol—20 mg or less of cholesterol and 2 grams or less of saturated fat per serving

- Low sodium—less than 140 mg of sodium per serving

- Reduced—at least 25% less per serving of the specified calories or nutrients compared to the regular variety of the food

- Light—1/3 fewer calories or 1/2 the fat of the regular variety

- Good source of—at least 10% to 19% of the Daily Value (DV) per serving of a specified nutrient

- Plus, more, added—at least 10% more of the DV for protein, vitamins, minerals, fiber and potassium per serving than the reference or original food

- High in, rich in, or excellent source of—contains 20% or more of the DV per serving of a specified nutrient

- High fiber—contain 5 grams or more of fiber per serving[3,4]

While not considered nutrient content claims here are some examples of food marketing terms found on food packaging:

- Organic, 100% organic, made with organic ingredients—meets the specific standards of the USDA's Organic Foods Production Act and the National Organic Program as being a food produced or grown without synthetic fertilizers or pesticides

- Natural—the food contains no artificial ingredients and a minimum amount of processing[5]

Daily Value (DV) is a term created to help consumers use food labels to plan their daily food intake. The percentage provides a guide to determine the percent one serving of that food contributes to the daily diet of a person eating 2000 calories per day. It helps consumers figure out if a food is too high or too low in a particular nutrient. For example, bread number 1 contains 25% of the DV for fiber per serving and bread number 2 contains 2% of the DV for fiber; bread number 1 is clearly the higher fiber bread choice.[3-5]

The nutrition facts label on foods lists both the nutrients and fiber we need to get enough of each day and those we should limit. Aim to get 100% of the DV for dietary fiber, vitamin A and C, calcium and iron each day. Limit sodium, total fat, cholesterol, and saturated fat intake to no more than 100% of the DV each day.

* * *

THE BIG CHICKEN DINNER: *Once upon a time I worked in the retail grocery industry. I loved my job. It was dynamic and fun. One day I was on a conference call along with several of its executives. During the call I heard it announced that the 'Healthy Low Carbo Chicken Dinner' would soon be rolled out across America in the deli section of our stores. The voice on the line described that the promotion would be complete with signage to possibly include the nutrition program logo. It just so happened that that was the program I was responsible for and this was the first I was hearing of the promotion.*

To the best of my recollections the dinner included creamed cauliflower, fried chicken, and some other high-fat food. When the voice finished with the description I found myself blurting out something along the lines of, "Hi, Anita here, this is the first I've heard of this promotion. I'm uncomfortable with this promotion using the nutrition program logo as that infers this deal is nutritious. If you insist on using it then I recommend you slap a neon sticker with 9-1-1 on each dinner sold because that's who our customers will need to call after they're done eating it. Better yet, let's change our promo signage to read 'the heart attack special.'"

Dead silence. I wasn't done. My finale was to point out the chances of lawsuits against us for lack of truth in advertising. As the story goes, I found out later the company's chief attorney just happened to be on that conference call. I was told later, after hearing my candid remarks, the attorney decided to investigate the possible legal backlash a promotion like this one could result in. Investigation completed he exercised sound judgment recommending the promotion be pulled. And it was. Bravo to the wise grocery chain and their legal counsel. Did you know that there is no regulation of the term healthy?

● ● ●

Since 1966 the FDA and other government entities have had their work cut out for them. In my humble opinion, these regulators have what I term a *Goldilocks and the Three Bears* approach to regulation system where a food product must measure up to strict requirements to gain permission to bear a nutrient content claim. The food product must be:

- Not too big: must not contain too much of a nutrient to harm you.

- Not too small: must meet specific nutrient requirements for each health claim, *e.g. folic acid and neural tube defects.*

- Just right: must be a good source or greater than or equal to 10% of the Daily Value for at least one nutrient (vitamin A, vitamin C, iron, calcium, protein or fiber), without fortification.

In the age of the organic food craze and legislation regulating trans fats in foods, I believe the sales of magic potions in a bottle or box continues. *Snake oil* and *magic elixirs* have been replaced in name only with fortified or enriched foods, dietary supplements, and gimmicks that promise magic results or your money back.

* * *

SNAKE OIL DEFINED: *A product that has been proven to not live up to the vendor's marketing hype. The term comes from the 1800s in which elixirs and potions of all kinds, even those that supposedly included real snake oil, were sold as a cure for everything that ailed a person. Since then efforts have been made to get the scientific truth out to the consumers without confusing us.*

* * *

Right Size Your Body

According to data from the National Health and Nutrition Examination Survey (NHANES) 2003-2006 and 2007-2008 over 66% of adults in the United States are overweight and over 33% of that group is obese. The major cause of being overweight or obese is simple, eating more calories than you burn. However, overweight and obesity can also be a side effect of taking certain medications, genetics, and the environment. Obesity creates its own risk factors which include:

- Type 2 diabetes
- Coronary heart disease
- High LDL, or lousy cholesterol
- Stroke
- Hypertension
- Non-alcoholic fatty liver disease

- Pancreatitis

- Gallbladder disease

- Osteoarthritis or degeneration of cartilage and bone of joints.

- Sleep apnea and other breathing problems

- Some forms of cancer such as breast, colorectal, endometrial, and kidney

- Complications of pregnancy[6]

You certainly do have control over right sizing your weight. *Yes, you do!* Overweight and obesity are preventable and/or treatable in most cases. According to the CDC overweight and obesity are both terms for ranges of weight that are greater than what is generally considered healthy for a given height. The terms also identify ranges of weight that have been shown to increase the likelihood of certain diseases and other health problems.[7] Weight is stated in terms of body mass index, or *BMI*. BMI is the relationship of weight to height taking into account gender. Years of statistics have shown that individuals whose weight fell within certain ranges were at a higher risk for disease and for morbidity (disease or illness) or mortality (death) because of their weight. A BMI of 18.5 to 24.9 is considered healthy. A person with a BMI of 25 to 29.9 is considered overweight. Obesity is defined when a person's BMI is greater than 30. The body mass index chart is useful for most adults.[8] While there is a separate BMI chart for children, Table 8.1 is lists an abbreviated version of an adult BMI chart.

Use Table 8.1 to determine your BMI. This table offers a sample of BMI measurements. First, find your height on the far left column. Next, move across the row to find your weight. Weight is measured with underwear but no shoes. Once you've found your weight, move to the very top of that column. This number is your BMI. If you don't see your height and/ or weight listed on this table, go to the NHLBI's complete Body Mass Index Table listed in Appendix C.

Table 8.1 Body Mass Index Values For Adults

Height	21	22	23	24	25	26	27	28	29	30	31
4'10"	100	105	110	115	119	124	129	134	138	143	148
5'0"	107	112	118	123	128	133	138	143	148	153	158
5'1"	111	116	122	127	132	137	143	148	153	158	164
5'3"	118	124	130	135	141	146	152	158	163	169	175
5'5"	126	132	138	144	150	156	162	168	174	180	186
5'7"	134	140	146	153	159	166	172	178	185	191	198
5'9"	142	149	155	162	169	176	182	189	196	203	209
5'11"	150	157	165	172	179	186	193	200	208	215	222
6'1"	159	166	174	182	189	197	204	212	219	227	235
6'3"	168	176	184	192	200	208	216	224	232	240	248

Source: US Department of Health and Human Services, National Institutes of Health, and National Heart, Lung, and Blood Institute. Available at: http://www.nhlbi.nih.gov/health/dci/Diseases/obe/obe_diagnosis.html. Accessed February 28, 2011.

It is important to remember that although BMI correlates with the amount of body fat, BMI does not directly measure body fat. As a result, some people, such as athletes, may have a BMI that identifies them as overweight even though they do not have excess body fat. For certain conditions, using the BMI to measure health as it relates to weight, may not be accurate or appropriate. If you are unsure check with your registered dietitian or physician.[7,8]

It's easy to gain weight one mouthful at a time. Signs of weight gain include: snug fitting and uncomfortable clothes, the scale shows a higher number, extra belly fat is accumulating and you can no longer bend over to tie your shoes because your stomach is in the way, you just can't move about as easily as before, or your size and inability to breathe may be interfering with your movement. The key is to take action as the first sign of unwanted weight gain.

* * *

FACT: *A waist measurement of greater than 35 inches for a woman and greater than 40 inches for a man increases risk of heart disease and other medical conditions related to obesity.*[8]

* * *

Butt and Gut Dropping Ideas

If you are not at a healthy weight or your desired weight I encourage you to get busy. The good news is that you can change what you weigh. Start by setting realistic goals that are measureable. A registered dietitian can help you in this process. If you are willing I guarantee the RD is ready. An RD will teach you life skills to lose weight and have fun in the process. *Yes, you will!* You didn't gain the weight overnight and will not and should not lose the unwelcome pounds overnight. Take small steps. Once you've reached each goal reward yourself with a non-food treasure. Retail therapy can work if you're able to stay within a budget.

If you use more calories than you eat you'll lose weight. This is accomplished by eating a balanced diet and being physically active. Cutting back on calories and changing your behavior can help you lose weight. To lose one to two pounds a week, adults should cut back their calorie intake by 500 calories a day and increase activity, calorie expenditure, by 500 calories.

- In general, eating 1,200 to 1,400 calories a day will help most women lose weight safely.

- In general, eating 1,500 to 1,800 calories a day will help most men lose weight safely. This calorie range is also suitable for women who weigh 165 pounds or more or who exercise routinely.

These calorie levels are a general guide and may need to be adjusted. Seek an RD's advice for the exact number of calories needed to reach your weight goal. Very low-calorie diets of less than 800 calories a day shouldn't be used unless your doctor is monitoring you.[9]

*   *   *

FACT: *Generally speaking a 500 calorie per day decrease in calorie intake can yield a 3500 calorie deficit which is equal to one pound of body fat or one pound loss per week. A safe weight loss program is usually a loss of no more than 2.5 pounds per week.*

*   *   *

For overweight children or teens, it's important to slow the rate of weight gain; however, reduced-calorie diets aren't advised. A child or adolescent should not go on a diet before consulting with the child's physician. Request that the physician refer you and your child to a registered dietitian with the skills to help you help your child. **Except in extreme cases, children shouldn't be on weight reduction diets at all.** Children should be allowed to grow into their weight, if they are overweight, not obese, and do not have underlying health conditions. Just make sure the food offered to your child is nutritious, in child proportions, and that they get plenty of exercise—at least one hour per day. Resist offering them sugary juice drinks as a substitute for soda pop and candy, *please.*

Bad habits die hard. Stay accountable for what, when, why, where, and how much you eat. An excellent tool for getting in touch with your inner eating is to keep a journal to help you track your eating activities. Just because you did not write it down, it does not mean you did not eat it! Many foods considered 'Free' do contain calories. No one is more responsible for your food choices and or amounts eaten than you.

By brushing your teeth right after you've eaten to get the taste of food out of your mouth you'll be less likely to snack between meals. If you can start with one of the following strategies each week, you'll be ahead while losing your behind:

- Clear food off counters to decrease temptation each time you walk by. The cookie you grab and chomp into each time you walk by could easily add up to a half-a-dozen before you know it.

- Fill your plate in the kitchen versus eating family-style where you can continue to replenish you plate without getting up from the table.

- Eat from a measuring cup, not from the bag when eating high-calorie, high-fat foods.

- Divide a bag of your favorite high-calorie, high-fat snacks into individual portions. Discipline yourself to only eat one portion.

- Wear your tightest outfit when dining out. It will keep you honest in the amount you eat. Wearing elastic or drawstring waist clothes can lead to overeating.

- Dine with people who you find pleasing to converse with. Why? Crabby people make you focus on the food and you eat more than usual as you're trying to avoid conversation.

Celebration Eating Strategies

It's easy to maintain a healthy body weight even when holidays and other celebrations roll around. Plan ahead and you can survive any celebration, from New Year's Eve to Christmas Day. You'll find each one of these tips works like a charm:

- Work party-going into your daily meal pattern by eating lighter and more nutritious foods at the festivities; offer to take a healthy food item, and make sure you do not go to the party hungry.

- Maintain a regular exercise routine throughout the holidays. Besides being an excellent stress-reliever, regular exercise will help keep off the extra "party pounds." Wake up early on party days and get plenty of exercise. This will help keep your mind right for eating healthy the day of the party.

- Limit alcohol intake. Alcohol naturally stimulates appetite, reduces inhibitions and can work against good judgment and your willpower to eat healthily. If you do decide to drink then alternate alcoholic beverages with non-alcoholic alternatives. Enjoy a tangy fruit juice spritzer, sparkling water, flavored teas or coffees. Need to just have something in your hand? Ginger ale or tonic water (diet is best) on the rocks with a twist of lemon or lime works great.

- Say goodbye to grazing and fill up on good conversation away from the fatty food section of the get-together. Before you go to a party, eat a low-fat snack like high-fiber cereal with nonfat milk or a piece of fresh fruit. These strategies can help to curb your appetite so you don't over-indulge.

- Take a nibble and leave the rest. If you try some food you've never eaten before and find you don't like it, gracefully set it back on your plate. Don't feel compelled to eat everything.

- Go with Holiday Hot House Cider, the recipe is listed under 'H' in Chapter 11, as a crowd pleaser. This can replace the cream-based or mocha hot drinks at your party. Doll it up a bit by naming it the *Hot House Special*. Piping hot mulled apple cider is an option for this simple delight garnished with a slice of orange or lemon.

- Go fat-free on beverages. Buy eggnog minus the fat and booze. That choice can cut as many as 300 calories per one cup serving.

- Evaporate the fat. Use fat-free or low-fat evaporated milk in recipes instead of the full-fat version. Typically there is little to no taste difference in the final product.

- Choose or offer dip with fruits, vegetables or pretzels. Cut up these natural favorites for handy scoopers to replace cheese trays and chip bowls. Less guilt and more fiber.

- Go sour on the cream. Instead of creamy-based dips for vegetables or pretzels, use low-fat ranch dressing, mustard, hummus, bean dip, or salsa. For cut-up fruits use low-fat yogurt, low-fat pudding, or cinnamon applesauce.

- Shake the salt. Experiment ahead of time on decreasing salt in your recipes. There is always enough salt in other party foods that will make up for it.

- Go lean on your meat. Use healthier cuts of meats that are naturally lower in fat. If you select beef go for round, loin or chuck cuts. Prime cuts are higher in fat, cost more and show-up with white waxy fat once at room temperature. Turkey or chicken breast meat is a sandwich favorite.

- Send leftovers home with your guests. If you do have high fat snacks at your party send your guests home with those leftovers. High-fat and high-sugar foods should be first in the must go goodie bags you send home with guests.

Right Size Your Activity Level

Physical activity is an under-rated natural antidepressant. Activity switches the brain from the right side (creative, artistic, limbic, and emotional) and to the left side (calculating, cortical, and active). How does being physically active help you overall? Personally, physical activity helps clear my head so I can think more clearly and positively impacts my physical, emotional, and spiritual well-being. It can do the same for you.

Of all the things that have helped me cope with stress and anxiety, exercise has always been my secret weapon. A common saying in the circles of the Twelve-Step recovery program is, *When I Got Busy, I Got Better.* The Twelve-Step program consists of twelve guiding steps and traditions to help a person overcome addiction, compulsion, codependency, or other behavioral problems. Originally proposed by Alcoholics Anonymous, the program has since been applied to other addictive behaviors. The saying about getting busy and getting better holds true regardless of your lifestyle. Exercise and other positive activities help the brain refocus on something positive, attainable and in the now. Along with helping you sleep better, getting your move on can help put whatever is bugging you into prospective.

Regardless of the time of year, activity or exercise needs to be a part of your daily routine. Being fit can help you:

- Reach your ideal weight and maintain it for a lifetime

- Improve your mood, reduce stress, and increase energy levels

- Reduce your risk of heart disease, cancer and diabetes

- Gain endurance and strength to do the things you want to do

- Improve bone strength, especially if you do aerobic, weight-bearing exercises such as walking, jogging, gardening or tennis

Aerobic activities increase your heart rate and make you sweat while non-aerobic activities such as watching TV, playing cards, computer games, talking on the telephone, generally do not.

All adults should get 30-60 minutes of planned exercise most days of the week. Children and teens should get a minimum of 60 minutes each day. Listed below are examples of the average calories burned during a variety of physical activities of 30 minutes in length. Figures in Table 8.2 are for a healthy 150-pound adult. A person weighing less will burn fewer calories and person weighing over 150 pounds will use more calories.[10]

Table 8.2 Estimated Calories Used During 30 Minutes of Selected Activities.

ACTIVITY	CALORIES USED
Walking (leisurely), 2 miles/hour	85
Garden work	135
Raking leaves	145
Walking (brisk) 4 miles/hour	170
Traditional dancing	190
Bicycling (leisurely), 10 miles/hour	205
Chopping wood	205
Ice skating, skiing, or sledding	240
Swimming laps, moderate exertion	240
Jogging 5 miles/hour	275

Source: US Department of Health and Human Services, National Institute of Health, National Heart, Lung, and Blood Institute. Available at: http://www.nhlbi.nih.gov/health/prof/heart/other/aian_manual/ak_manual.pdf. Accessed October 30, 2010.

Physical activity positively impacts heart health, muscle, strength and bone health. Being physically active on a regular basis helps build your physical strength, endurance, flexibility, and balance. Here are some basic guidelines to get you started:

- First, pick an activity that you find easy, fun and interesting and then allow enough time in your schedule to do it regularly.

- Drink plenty of water before, during and after exercise.

- Eat a healthy diet with plenty of complex carbohydrate for fast energy.

- Gear up with appropriate footwear, clothing, and protective gear.

- Rest enough between activity sessions for your body to recover.

- Start slowly with 10–15 minutes per day to build endurance. If you are not used to exercising, start slowly building on your success. If you overdo it in the beginning you'll be less likely to want to continue because all you will remember is that you were so sore the next day that you could hardly function. *Easy does it.*

- Invest in a step counter or pedometer to wear throughout the day to track of how far you walk just doing normal daily activities.

- Log your time, distance, heart rate, and mood after each session to track your progress.

What you eat, how much you move, and how you handle stress will determine how successful you'll be at obtaining and maintaining optimum health and healthy weight.

Into Action

We learned in Chapter 2 that water is a key nutrient essential for normal body function. This is also true for any kind of physical activity. Regardless of your level of physical activity or athletic competition follow these general hydration guidelines:

- Drink water and other fluids throughout the day to keep your body well hydrated.

- Start every exercise session already well hydrated.

- Sip on water during exercise to replace fluids lost by sweating.

- Water is the fluid of choice for short duration of low to moderate intensity activity lasting less than 60 minutes.[11]

- Rehydrate after exercise to replace any weight you lost during exercise. A good rule of thumb is to drink two cups of water for every pound lost during exercise.

Know that bottled water has no significant nutritional advantage over tap water, plus the plastic or glass clutters up the environment. Unless you're outside the United States, you can choose to drink only bottled water. Some bottled waters are from natural springs claiming magical results. Some are filtered to remove undesirable flavors. Others may have come from the tap. Yes. The same water source as comes out of your kitchen faucet; it isn't illegal to sell water bottled from a tap water source, in fact, some companies have been found to do so.[12]

* * *

WATER MONEY: *If you drink eight cups (64 ounces) of water per day at $1 per 16 ounce bottle you can save at least $1460 per year by drinking tap water. Make your own tap water better tasting by passing it through a filter, or draw a pitcher from the tap and place it in the refrigerator for a couple hours; you will notice its flavor is enhanced.*

* * *

Generally speaking the water systems in the United States, where water utilities treat nearly 34 billion gallons of water every day, provide safe drinking water. In the United States and Canada, the total miles of water pipeline and aqueducts equal approximately one million miles; enough to circle the globe 40 times.[13] These same statistics aren't necessarily true for all countries. If your physical activity takes you to outside the United States, it is good to know where your drinking water comes from and if and how it is treated. When in doubt about water, drink it bottled.

Sports Drinks or Not

The sports and 'energy' drink industry is a multi-million dollar business. These products contain mostly water, vitamins and minerals, and sometimes sweeteners. If you do moderate to high intensity activities for over an hour a sports or energy drink may be beneficial particularly for the purposes of replacing electrolytes and carbohydrates. The optimal sugar concentration for quick absorption is 6–8% carbohydrate.[11] Here are examples of energy drinks and the percent of sugar in each:

- Gatorade™- 6.5%

- PowerAde™- 8%

- Regular cola—10%

- Red Bull™- 11%

- Apple juice- 12%[14]

Any liquid with a sugar content over 8% is more likely to cause stomach distress such as cramping and diarrhea. The gut can't rapidly absorb sugar at such a concentration rate. Regardless of the type of fluid you drink or your activity level, water is the most essential nutrient for good body function and to help fight off disease and infection.

The body depends on the electrolytes sodium, potassium, calcium, magnesium, chloride and phosphate to maintain optimal body chemistry. Be sure to replenish these electrolytes lost during physical activity by consuming foods with high water contents rich in these minerals. Some food and beverage sources high in electrolytes include:

- Potassium—highest amounts found in fruits and vegetables especially bananas, citrus fruits, raisins, soybeans and potatoes

- Sodium—highest amounts found in salt, salted foods, soups and vegetable juices

- Calcium- highest amounts found in dairy products (regardless of fat content) and some vegetables

See Chapter 2 for more information on each mineral and its related food sources.

Energy Sources for Activity

Picking the right foods that render the most energy is important regardless of your activity level. Carbohydrates are the first responders to the body's need for energy during exercise. Protein and fat are not nearly as efficient as carbohydrate in providing energy for running, skiing, hiking or other types of activities.

Carbohydrates are broken down by the body into glucose and provide a quick and primary source of energy. Unlike fat, carbohydrate cannot be stored in large amounts by the body. When stored, carbohydrate is found in the muscles and liver in the form of glycogen.

Carbohydrates power the body to do everything from maintaining good heart function to hiking to the top of Mount Whitney or the bottom of the Grand Canyon. Depending on how long you plan to be moving down the trail, around the gym or down the lane I recommend taking along twice the amount of carbohydrates you plan on consuming.

If you're headed out to perform an endurance activity choose foods that provide quick energy without much fiber or fat. Why? Too much fiber will lend to bowel activity and that means using a toilet. Fiber is great but easy does it on high fiber foods for marathon running, distance biking, and hiking. Select foods from the grain/cereal, fruit and vegetable group as the mainstay of your food supply, not as snacks to munch on while moving. Hit the trail with the following healthy food ideas for your next fitness experience. These are some tasty tried and true pre-exercise and post-exercise healthy snack ideas:

- Whole-grain bagel with (natural) peanut butter and yogurt.

- Thin-crust pizza with green peppers.

- Granola with low-fat milk and banana.

- Trail mix with nuts and dried fruit.

- Instant oatmeal made with low-fat milk.

- Bran or corn muffin with egg whites and salsa.

- Fig bars with (natural) peanut butter and juice.

- Take a carton of ultra-pasteurized boxed milk along on ice in a cooler and drink it cold at the end of the trail or finish line.

From homemade granola to crispy apples each hiker has his or her own favorites to pack. Granny Smith or Fuji apples and homemade granola chucked full of raisins, dried apricots and apples, unsalted almonds and walnuts are my family favorites. Try the Walk the Trail Mix recipe in Chapter 11 for an easy to make and tasty trail snack.

A chocolate bar with almonds provides carbohydrates from the sugar, fat from the chocolate and nuts, and a dab of protein from almonds sprinkled in the bar. A chocolate bar chucked full of almonds is a favorite to bring along to nibble on during a hike, if the weather is cool. A bite of a chocolate bar gives a bit of caffeine and sweetness for quick energy, but don't overdo it!

Long Haul Foods

When planning for overnight activities like hiking, biking, or camping for several days this handy grocery list will provide some helpful hints. Tailor it to your likes and needs by including some of your favorite packable foods and beverages. Here's a food shopping list to get you started in planning for your next outing:

- Fresh apples, oranges and potatoes.

- Peanut butter (in a plastic jar).

- Dried soup, noodles and rice.

- Nuts, dried fruits, and food bars.

- Dehydrated foods such as beans or those purchased from a camping supply store.

- Powdered milk and 100% fruit juice.

- Powdered mixtures for pancakes or biscuits.

- Beef jerky and other dried meats.

- Vacuum foil packed salmon, tuna, ham, chicken, and beef.

Pack like items together in plastic bags. Example: pack dried rice, pasta, and baking mixes in the same bag. Whether an afternoon outing or two day overnight hike, choose foods light enough to carry in your backpack and that can transport safely.

Canned foods are convenient to just open and heat up on the campfire but make for a heavier load. Most outings that involve an all day activity and the preparation of one or two meals may call for some cooking gear. Ultra light weight cooking gear can fit the bill and not load you down.

Be sure to incorporate food safety when handling food as foodborne illness is never a welcome guest at any picnic or camping trip. *Keep hot foods hot and cold foods cold* is the golden rule which is always followed by *keep it clean* to make sure your adventures make for only good memories. The USDA Food Safety and Inspection Service has abundant information on food safety and why it's important, for your next outing. For more on food safety refer to the *resource section* under *food safety, labeling and advertising* in the back of the book.[15]

A Word or Two About Stress

There is that split second pause we experience when faced with a choice do I go through the yellow light or stop? Do I eat French fries or a salad? Should I add cream or skim milk to my cup of coffee or drink it black? Making healthy food choices consistently can help you feel better, have more energy, and armor yourself for handling stress more efficiently.[16]

Notice I am not requiring you to be boringly perfect! All foods can fit in a healthy diet. If food *IS* your booze…like vodka is booze to the alcoholic…then accept the addiction and resist the compulsion. Ditch the guilt and get on with your life.

What is driving your desire for unhealthy behaviors? Let's start with your current stress level. Do you work too much, exercise too little, sleep poorly, and eat whatever is convenient? The answer to some or all of the above may be sometimes *yes* and other times *no*. How you cope with stress can be a deal breaker for the onset of chronic disease. People who have an outlet to blow off steam through physical activity or other healthy activities have an edge over those who stuff stress until they have a heart attack, stroke or high blood pressure. Deal with your stress or I guarantee you it will deal with you.

Welcome to the human race. And it does seem like a race a good deal of the time. Ask yourself these four questions:

Am I hungry? Learn how to discern if you're experiencing real hunger or perceived hunger. Before you grab something to eat figure out if you are truly hungry or just bored. Are you thirsty rather than hungry? Slow down and sit down; with your mouth closed let your tongue rest relaxed, sinking low to the floor of your mouth. Close your eyes. Take a deep breath. Hold it for a count of three. Exhale slowly through pursed lips. Relax. Repeat this three times. Before you open your eyes ask your tummy if it's hungry. If the answer is *no* then get your move on. If the answer is *yes* to the above question, eat something healthy with protein, complex carbohydrates, and a small amount of healthy fat. Try a glass of skim milk and a slice of whole grain toast with a dab of chunky peanut butter, or an apple with a dab of almond butter.[16] The point is to not run on empty—the body needs a consistent flow of energy to keep all its systems running optimally.

Hunger, anger, loneliness, exhaustion, and being a couch potato are sometimes excuses for why folks turn to food for comfort. Being tired is often rationalization for consuming excess amounts of caffeine or what

I label as *liquid stress* and alcohol or *liquid depression*. Left unchecked, these behaviors may become your enemies over the long term.

Sometimes when my day feels out of whack and it's not even mid-morning, I make the conscious decision to start my day over. You can, too. If it wasn't for this option I may have found myself writing this book behind bars or while sitting in one. Begin with the food you eat. Step away from the coffee maker, pour a tall glass of water and eat a handful of almonds or baby carrots and a stick of string cheese—you will feel your body switch into a more efficient gear.

Am I angry? Raging at a fly that keeps buzzing past you or screaming at the birds for tweeting too loudly may mean you're getting a bit edgy. If so, use this affirmation technique I learned from Howard Liebgold, M.D., a physiatrist and an expert at understanding and treating anxiety, panic, phobias and obsessive compulsive disorders. Take a deep breath, count to three and exhale slowly through pursed lips. Repeat this twice more. Ask yourself what is happening this very second. Then say to yourself, "I will handle it" to whatever the stress is. Stay in the moment and determine what the situation is and find a way to constructively deal with it in the now. You may need to find a short, simple activity to help you clear your head before tackling the situation head on. Take a short walk, do some breathing exercises, take out the trash, do math in your head, and count to ten. Avoiding the situation will only make it grow larger, if not in reality, at least in your mind.[16,17]

Getting angry is a normal part of life. What you do with that emotion will be the difference between prison time and going to the spa for a massage. Anger and frustration may be generated from unfulfilled hopes and dreams, fear, pain, or hurt. Carrying around these emotions like a bright blinking light or white-hot coal will diminish your chances for happiness and peace. It's like the old saying—taking a dose of poison and then waiting for the other person to die. Anger only hurts you.

Do not give your power away to whomever or whatever is making you angry. Write down your feelings and then get on with your day. Talk to a trusted friend, go on a run, punch a punching bag—or try thanking the situation for teaching you another one of life's lessons. Really mad? Write it down on a strip of masking tape and stick it on the bottom of your shoe then walk around on it until you're over the feeling. My first and last advice to you when you are harboring resentment is to pray for the person or situation you're resenting or angry with. This works like a charm for me.

Am I lonely? Are you the only one invited to the pity party you've decided to throw in your honor? Do you look back and regret yesterday, instead of looking at today and tomorrow with hope? If so, make a list of the things you like to do like a "do before I kick the bucket list," and then one by one, do each one. Share some of these activities with someone else. Don't isolate yourself. If we were meant to be alone there wouldn't have been over nearly seven billion other people created to live on Earth with us.[16]

Adopt a pet, volunteer at the local animal shelter or visit some seniors at a nursing home. Offer to walk your neighbor's dog. Pick up the newspaper in front of your neighbor's house or apartment and place it on their doorstep. Take yourself out on a date to the local movie house or go get a massage. Be kind to yourself.[16]

Am I tired? I don't know about you, but I am a workaholic. I have learned that I am usually worn out at the end of my day because I don't know when to stop and say "NO!" Or I may be worn out from spending my day nursing resentment, or from trying to live someone else's life for them. Am I trying to force solutions to my own problems? Or trying to solve someone else's problems? And I know I am not alone in my thinking and behavior.

Let's start with: do you take your job home? Literally, do you bring home work in the evenings or off-duty time to complete? I hereby give you permission to stop doing this. I came to the realization that the more extra hours I worked over my paid hours lowered my hourly pay rate. And it lowered my self-esteem in the process. Sometimes extra work is unavoidable and a part of being a professional but regular take-home work isn't healthy nor will it make you happy. All work and no play can lead to a very stressful life.[16]

Self-care is a discipline. Teach and allow yourself to stop working at a certain time of day—and stick to it. Being overly tired may lead to consuming food, drink or drugs that interrupt the sleep process. Don't consume substances such as caffeine, alcohol or stimulants that will keep you awake when you ought to be sleeping. If you can't rest or sleep because you're a light sleeper or someone snores, buy some earplugs.[16] Daily exercise may also help you sleep more soundly. To get the best sleep results experts recommend a cool, dark, and quiet environment.

Can't rid yourself of the source of the noise when you're trying to sleep? Deep breathing may help you fall asleep. See a healthcare professional like a physician or psychotherapist who can help you if the problem persists. Snoring can be a sign of sleep apnea, which if untreated, can lead to lack of oxygen and in rare cases can even lead to death.[16] From a practical standpoint, if it's your partner in a relationship then moving out of the room instead of moving out of the house is always an option. This can be a very effective stress management tool for both the relationship and you.

You Are What You Eat

To help cope with stress do yourself a favor and start your day by eating breakfast. Keep in mind a day started with a balanced breakfast followed by eating regularly keeps your blood sugar at optimal levels keeping you calm and relaxed. Over the past 20 plus years of dietetics practice here are some of the common excuses for not eating breakfast that I have heard:

- Eating breakfast makes me gain weight.

- I'm not hungry when I get up in the morning.

- Just the thought of food before Noon gags me.

- I wake up too late to eat breakfast.

- I don't have time, I'm too busy.

Any excuse will do when you don't want to do something. You'll be more productive and less moody by simply adding breakfast to your day. Eating breakfast helps to maintain a healthy body weight. Remember that a healthy diet begins with adequate amounts of protein, carbohydrate, fat, vitamins, minerals, and fluids.[16] Here are some meal ideas to get you started:

- Oatmeal made with 1% milk or fortified soy milk; whole wheat toast topped with strawberry jam; a medium banana.

- Blueberry pancakes topped with blueberry syrup; fruit salad; 1% milk.

- Egg pita (two scrambled eggs with low-fat cheese and salsa inside a whole-wheat pita); fresh fruit salad; cranberry juice.

Research has repeatedly shown that students who eat breakfast are more attentive in class, behave better, perform better in their studies, are less tardy, and do better on tests than those students who don't eat breakfast.[18] Eating breakfast fuels your brain for optimal functioning. If you wait until lunch to eat, you have gone about 15 hours without nourishment. So break the fast. Your brain and body need ongoing nourishment to help you think clearly, stay perky, and maintain an adequate energy level.

Recipe to Be Right Sized

- Follow the peaceful way. Strive for activities and behaviors that bring you calm, serenity, and positive results.

- Set measurable, realistic, and achievable goals.

- Right size your food choices and portion sizes.

- Right size your body by maintaining a healthy weight.

- Right size your fitness level with at least 30—60 minutes of physical activity daily.

- Take a *before* and *after* picture of yourself to compare the new you.

- Don't skip breakfast.

- Plan meals ahead of time.

- Be sure to include foods rich in vitamins A, C and E in your daily food plan. These nutrients are paramount to good health and optimal immunity.

- Limit or omit alcohol and caffeine intake.

- Follow the peace when eating—anything, at any time. Take a break to dine in a peaceful environment as often as possible.

- Limit high-fat and high-calorie comfort foods to once or twice a month.

- Get regular, uninterrupted sleep.

- If you lapse, don't relapse. Get right back on track and do not beat yourself up for straying from your plan.

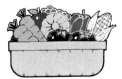

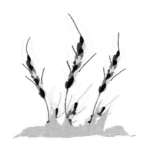

NINE

HAPPY HOE DOWN

Gardening, starting with home-grown luscious produce is a wonderful way to become self-sustaining. It's good for your body, mind, and soul.

Grow Your Own

My garden is an expression of my food preferences and my confidence in Mother Nature's abilities to nourish me. The urban farming movement includes good, old fashioned gardening that's been around since the Garden of Eden. If you like to think growing your own food is a new concept and that motivates you to eat healthier, then get busy gardening.

Regardless of your gardening experience and skill, the ritual of preparing, planting, watering, weeding, and harvesting your own produce will not fail to give you a sense of fulfillment and oneness with nature. Deferring to nature builds patience, humility, and self esteem. An appreciation of "perfect timing" gives a sense of having complied with the natural order of the universe. It is always worth the effort.

Gardening is great for the **body** providing exercise, fresh air, perspiration that helps cleanse the body, builds flexibility, and strengthens your muscles and bones.

Gardening is good for the **mind** by relieving stress and helping you focus on the prospect of something positive. It's the opportunity to hoe up the ground versus clobber our enemies, keeping us out of jail and off the national news. Gardening will provide time to change gears as the brain shifts from the limbic or creative, artistic, emotional right-side to the activity focused, calculating, or cortical left-side.

Gardening is good for the **soul** providing a reconnection with nature and its seasons. There is something about gardening that seems holy. It *is* holy to me. It's an act of faith that if I do my part Mother Nature will do hers.

● ● ●

DOWN THE YELLOW BRICK PATH: *I can easily recreate in my memory strutting down the dirt path to our garden, salt shaker in hand. I was on my way to devour a couple big, red ripe tomatoes. The sight of the shiny, plump red tomatoes hanging like fat Christmas balls from the dozen or two of vines made it hard to decide which one to snatch as my snack. I'd use the garden hose to rinse the tomato with a squirt of water. Then snip the skin of the tomato with my teeth to make a wet spot where the salt would stick to the shiny gem. A dash of salt in the wet spot and the feasting began.*

● ● ●

The Garden Groove

Gardening requires sunlight, space to plant, basic watering, weeding, and patience. Follow these basic guidelines to make your first gardening experience a successful and happy one.

Location, location, location is not just the mantra recited by realtors. Gardeners say it, too. The most important first step is the selection of the right location for your garden. Match the plant to its best environment planting the right plant in the right place at the right time. Adequate sunlight, rich soil with good drainage, and good access to your source of water are vital. Let's get started by making sure we know the following:

- Sunlight. The garden term full sun means a minimum of 6 hours of sunlight a day. If the seed package instructions require full sun and plenty of water to grow provide both. If the planting instructions indicate *partial sun* means 4 to 6 hours of direct sunlight. *Shade* means the absence of direct sun.[1]

- Timing. Know your *hardiness zone*. This USDA developed planting gauge is a geographic guide based on winter minimum temperatures throughout the US. Use this map to determine the geographic zone where you live. Plant the types of plants that thrive in your zone. Access the hardiness zone map that includes details for its use online at: http://www.usna.usda.gov. Or, contact your local library, county Cooperative Extension agent or local nursery for this information. While there are other planting guides available I recommend starting with the USDA Plant Hardiness Zone map. See the *resource section* under *gardening and farming* for more information.

- Planting guidance. Always plant the seed or seedling according to package directions or plant tag information for sun, planting depth, spacing between seeds or plants, and watering guidance. Seeds and seedlings can be easily dropped to the right depth in prepared soil when the planting time is right. Typically the smaller the seed, the closer to the surface of the soil it should be planted.

- Soil. By definition, the terms *prepared soil* and *healthy soil* mean the ground is dug up and capable of nourishing a seed or seedling into a plant that bears fruit or vegetable. If your soil is average in richness (weeds or plants grow in the soil now), add a couple inches of compost or top soil. Work the ground with a hoe and rake until the old soil and new soil are evenly combined.[2]

● ● ●

COMPOST COMMENTS: *Plant remains and other once-living materials can be composted to make an earthy, dark, crumbly substance that is wonderful for enriching garden soil. Composting allows you to recycle yard and kitchen waste, and is one way to help decrease the amount of garbage unnecessarily sent to landfills for disposal. It's easy to learn how to compost. Refer to the resource section under gardening and farming for more on composting.*

● ● ●

- Watering. Moisture is essential for nearly all types of plant growth. The right amount of water is basic to optimal growth and development of your garden. This is true for grouping plants with like moisture needs together in one location. The basic watering methods include watering by hand, sprinkler, soaker hose, or drip irrigation. The first two methods are good choices for container gardens, hanging plants, newly planted seed beds, and hard to reach areas. Sprinklers work best for watering large areas. A soaker hose looks like a regular garden hose but is made of a permeable material that allows water to seep out of it directly into the ground. Drip irrigation is a low water pressure method of watering that allows water to pass through small holes in narrow plastic piping or plastic tubing either above or below ground and is usually permanently setup and left that way to use in subsequent planting seasons. Learn your city's rules on watering and whether it is in drought conditions. Water late at night or early morning to help lower evaporation. Always conserve water when possible.[2,3]

- Location alternatives. Consider raised beds if the location you've selected for your garden has less than ideal soil. Raised beds are easily installed by building up rich soil in a three (or more) sided box above ground level.[2] I planted a garden using this method when I lived in the Mojave Desert with great results.

      ●   ●   ●

DIRT CHEAP: *Aim to get the best price on any soil you buy. Why? Because I am genetically frugal and because the less money you spend on your garden project the lower your overhead. This means better sustainability and independence from of the grocery store. In reality, gardening can save money on food.*

      ●   ●   ●

Pesty Concerns

Healthy plants that flourish tend to have fewer pest and disease problems. Even when these are present, healthy plants stand up better than those suffering from being planted in the wrong place or wrong conditions.

When insects invite themselves into your garden don't automatically reach for pesticides and chemicals. When used incorrectly, pesticides can pollute water and kill both beneficial and harmful insects. Natural alternatives prevent this from happening and can save you money. Consider using natural alternatives for chemical pesticides such as non-detergent insecticidal soaps, garlic, hot pepper sprays, or a forceful stream of water to dislodge insects.

Consider using plants that naturally repel insects. Table 9.1 lists the plants that use their own chemical defense systems to help keep unwanted insects away from your garden when planted among flowers and vegetables.[4]

Table 9.1 Natural Pest Repellents

Pest	Plants
Ant	mint, tansy, pennyroyal
Aphid	mint, garlic, chives, coriander, anise
Bean Leaf Beetle	potato, onion, turnip
Colorado Potato Bug	green beans, coriander, nasturtium
Cucumber Beetle	radish, tansy
Flea Beetle	garlic, onion, mint
Imported Cabbage Worm	mint, sage, rosemary, hyssop
Japanese Beetle	garlic, larkspur, tansy, rue, geranium
Leaf Hopper	geranium, petunia
Mexican Bean Beetle	potato, onion, garlic, radish, petunia, marigolds
Mice	onion
Root Knot Nematode	French marigolds
Slugs	prostrate rosemary, wormwood
Spider Mite	onion, garlic, cloves, chives
Squash Bug	radish, marigolds, tansy, nasturtium
Stink Bug	radish
Thrips	marigolds
Tomato Hornworm	marigolds, sage, borage
Whitefly	marigolds, nasturtium

Source: US Department of Agriculture, Natural Resource Conservation Service. Home and garden tips: lawn and garden care—alternatives to pesticides and chemicals. Natural Resources Conservation Service. Available at: http://www.nrcs.usda.gov/feature/highlights/homegarden/lawn.html. Accessed February 2, 2011.

Critter Control

If you have problems with critters (cats, dogs, deer, birds and the like) helping themselves to your crop or relieving themselves on your soil then a fence or netting as a barrier is a good idea. Save the branches of your rose bush prunings and lay them out in the rows in your garden where the varmints enter. The naturally thorny branches will act as a barrier to unwanted guests.

* * *

WARNING: *Poisoning a critter is never the right answer when trying to solve invasion problems. Contact your local city animal control department for assistance on critter removal.*

* * *

Shoebox Gardening

Start gardening small by planting a lettuce garden in a shoebox. Line the shoebox with foil that you've poked little holes in with a toothpick or fork to allow water to drain out the bottom. Loosely fill the box with potting soil. Sit the box on a pan to catch excess water. Gently scatter some lettuce seeds into the soil at the depth indicated on the label, usually about 1/8th inch. Cover the seeds with soil. Usually the smaller the seed the less soil needed to cover it. If you plant a seed too deep its initial burst of sprout will fail to reach the surface to soak up the sun.

Sprinkle water on the soil until wet but not flooded. Overwatering will waterlog the soil and seeds may not sprout. Place the container near a window where it can be in the warmth and light of full sun. Lettuce requires full sun to grow. The seeds will take a few days to germinate and then should sprout above the soil. Once the lettuce gets to be about three to five (3-5) inches tall harvest with a scissors. Rinse off dirt and debris from the leaves, dab dry with a clean dish towel, and then chill in the refrigerator until crisp and serve in a salad.

Congratulations. Now you're ready to branch out to a larger chunk of ground to sow your seeds.

● ● ●

TOMATO TRIVIA: *Tomatoes are botanically a fruit and legally a vegetable. In a tariff dispute in the late 1800s a gang of attorneys decided it would be a vegetable.*

● ● ●

Progress—Not Perfection

Don't let it bother you if things don't turn out perfect the first planting season. If something sprouts from the spot where you planted the seed and it is green, you're a success. Have you ever seen a tree growing from a crack in the sidewalk? That's proof positive nature has a mind of its own and always gets the last word.

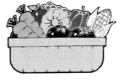

Seed—Seedling Selection

Here is a list of some seeds and seedlings that are easy to grow along with the major nutrients found in the food these produce.

Seed & Seedlings*	Nutrient
Corn	selenium, folate, thiamin
Onions	vitamin C, folate
Garlic	vitamin B6, vitamin C, calcium
Potatoes	potassium, selenium, vitamin B6
Turnips	vitamin C
Spinach	beta-carotene, vitamin C, iron, magnesium, vitamin E
Broccoli	beta-carotene, vitamin C, folate
Lettuce	vitamin C, beta-carotene,
Tomatoes	vitamin C, lycopene
Radishes	vitamin C, folate
Beets	vitamin C, lycopene
Zucchini	vitamin C, folate
Hot peppers	vitamin C, beta-carotene, vitamin B6, folate
Bell peppers	vitamin C, beta-carotene
Strawberries	vitamin C, lycopene, potassium
Peas	vitamin C, folate, thiamin, iron
Pumpkin	vitamin C, beta-carotene, folate
Swiss chard	vitamin C, beta-carotene, calcium, iron

*Check the USDA Plant Hardiness Zone map for details.

The Garden Pilot Project

Moving from a shoebox garden to an actual garden plot allows more space to sow seeds and plant seedlings into the earth. Here is a review of what you'll need to do the job:

- Sunshine

- Space

- Seeds or seedlings

- Nutrient rich soil

- Fertilizer and food that are organic, *green* or otherwise environmentally friendly type is best

- Water based on seed or seedling watering directions or guidance

- Timing based on plant hardiness zone guidance

- Tools including a *hoe* for chopping up the soil, covering seeds, and weeding; a sturdy *rake* for preparing the soil and breaking apart large clods of dirt; a *garden fork* and a *spade* to till the soil and add organic matter or compost to the dirt; a *bucket* and *watering can* to gently water new seedlings and seeds; *row markers* to identify what's planted where; *string* to make straight rows; and a *ruler* for accurate planting depth and distance between seeds, seedlings, and rows.

Always take the time to follow the seed package directions. Use the resources provided for online and phone support. You can also e-mail me with your questions and comments at info@foodfieldtofork.com.

* * *

GARDENER SHOCK: *I could hardly believe the first time I saw a single seedling of lettuce being sold at a local or chain nursery for a dollar or maybe two. I'd think to myself, "don't these folks know all they have to do is drop a seed in the ground, water it,*

let the sun shine on it and in a few days, voila—a seedling will
appear?" I promise you, with healthy soil, water, seed or seedling,
sun, and some tender loving care you can grow your own.

●   ●   ●

Gardening Health and Safety Tips

Keep your health in mind by gearing up to protect your body from the elements. From head-to-toe invest in the following to help protect your body as you garden:

- Sunscreen with a rating of SPF 45 or greater.

- Wide-brimmed hat (straw breathes well and is inexpensive) or cap.

- Safety goggles or sunglasses to protect your eyes for the sun's rays.

- Protect against diseases spread by mosquitoes and ticks by wearing insect repellent that contains DEET, long sleeves and long pants.

- Gardening gloves for protection against friction or unwanted soiling of your hands.

- Sturdy boots or shoes (leather or rubber materials are more water-resistant and protective than canvas or plastic).[5]

●   ●   ●

BEAUTY TIP: *Instantly treat your hands and cuticles to a hot oil treatment while gardening. In a pair of disposable gloves pour one tablespoon of vegetable oil into each glove. Slip on the gloves and massage the oil up and down your hand from the finger tips to your palms. Slip your gardening gloves over the latex gloves. When done gardening, remove both sets of gloves and note that* *all of the oil has been absorbed into your hands and cuticles. A slick beauty tip.*

● ● ●

Be a Petal Pusher—Edible Flowers

Incredible, edible flowers can be grown without the use of pesticides and make for some pretty fancy dining. Edible flowers are elegant additions to salads and as garnishes for a wide variety of other culinary dishes. Check to make sure the flowers you've chosen to consume are safe to eat. Contact the commercial ornamental and consumer horticulture Cooperative Extension agent in your county or use the online link http://www.ces.ncsu.edu for an extensive list of edible flowers.

More Advice

I love the friendly and helpful places where I can get my questions answered without opening my wallet called local libraries. Libraries can be accessed online, by telephone or in person. Government resources available include university and Cooperative Extension offices, USDA, FDA, and the National Agriculture Library. Usually free or at minimal cost to users these are great resources at your disposal.

The *gardening and farming* references in the *resource section* provides additional gardening information. Businesses specializing in seeds, plants, and gardening gadgets often have valuable ideas on gardening. Gardening magazines and gardening books you can borrow from the public library or buy at a newsstand are also good sources of information. Never give up before your questions are answered.

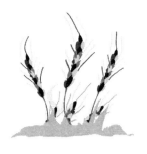

TEN

MY KITCHEN —MY KINGDOM

C avemen and cowboys cooked over campfires in the middle of the wilderness. So can you. Cooking can bring you comfort, joy and a sense of accomplishment. Using recipes that match and slightly stretch your cooking skills will move you closer to becoming a great cook.

The Cooking

If you can read and are willing to learn, you can learn to cook. If you already know how to cook my hope is this section will inspire you to cook more often.

Cooking is a verb. It means action. Cooking is accomplished when heat is applied to food. Examples include boiling, steaming, baking, broiling, and stir-frying. A recipe is the roadmap used to prepare food. A book of recipes with food preparation information is called a cookbook.

* * *

THE CIA: *Cooking is both an art and a science. In the mid-1990s I was a student at the Culinary Institute of American (CIA) in Hyde Park, NY for a course dedicated to cooking with the seasons. The CIA opened my eyes to the art of cooking. Our chef instructor reminded us often that the CIA graduated good cooks, not chefs. Chef is a title to be earned from hard work and repeated success. Our chef taught me about striving for* **mise en place,** *French for everything in place. The CIA taught me that for the best flavor and economy it's important to cook with the seasons.*

* * *

According to culinary historians, Archestratus, an Ancient Greek poet from Sicily may have written the first cookbook in the mid 4th century BC. Many of the basics we use in cooking methods today are the same as those used in ancient times. This is especially true about the similarities between the use of herbed vinegars and oil seasonings then and now.

The Recipe

Are you new to the kitchen and a bit intimidated or made nervous by the idea of learning to cook? Start getting into the mood by taking a long look through a very basic cookbook. Start with simple recipes having five or less ingredients.

Make your first stop the local library with a visit to their cookbook collection. Check out a couple cookbooks the librarian recommends as favorites of the cookbook crowd. The librarian may also be familiar with popular websites where you can find recipes online. Being a brave soul to have made it this far you're a shoe in to be successful at preparing a simple recipe.

Follow these easy guidelines when selecting a cookbook. Ideally, each recipe will have:

- Clear, easy to read step-by-step directions

- Pictures of how-to techniques and the finished product

- Basic definitions or descriptions of culinary terms used

- Nutritional analysis of the recipe

- Optional: CD or DVD tutorials on recipe preparation, list of appliances, pots, pans, and utensils needed to prepare recipes

If you are a beginner, consider enrolling in a locally taught cooking class designed for kitchen newbies. In a hurt-so-good sort of way, *misery really does love company.* Your community adult school and some cooking stores may have cooking classes for free or at a minimal cost. Also see the *resource section* because many of the websites I've listed contain recipe sections especially the *food industry* references.

The Tools

Besides a cookbook, the tools and equipment used during cooking should work correctly, be durable and heat resistant, but *not be costly.* Having the right tools on hand and using them will improve your odds of success. Second-hand stores and garage sales are great places to pick up some of these items for cheap.

- Measuring cups in 1 cup, 1/2 cup, 1/3 cup, 1/4 cup units

- Measuring spoons in 1 tablespoon, 1 teaspoon, 1/2 teaspoon, 1/4 teaspoon, 1/8 teaspoon increments

- Large mixing spoons and a sharp knife

- Oven thermometer, preferably the hanging type with an easy to read gauge

- Pocket food thermometer to check for the proper internal temperatures of cooked and chilled food

- A non-porous cutting board that can be washed in hot soapy water or the dishwasher

- An apron to protect your clothing from the food and vice versa

- At least one 3-quart saucepan and 8-quart stock pot

- At least one 1-quart and 3-quart bowls and a cookie sheet

- An electric hand mixer

- A stove, preferably with an oven and broiler

- Patience, concentration, and resilience

Apply *mise en place* throughout your cooking experience. Before you get started read your recipe through completely to make sure you have the right utensils and then gather them together to save time during the real-time recipe preparation. Just saying the words mise en place will make you feel more confident. Use it on your guests. Julia Child, the famous culinary goddess would be proud of you.

* * *

BENVENUTI: *Benvenuti means welcome in Italian. During a two year military tour on the island of Sicily, Italy I lived with a Sicilian family in a casa above the rustic village near Catania. This couple was the purest of the Sicilians from their faith to their food. Robust and passionate, they loved great food, great wine and generously welcomed us into their home. Thanks, Maria for teaching me to cook Sicilian-style. It was here that I was able to change what I thought I could not, my intolerance to foods made with onions or cooked tomatoes. I believe it was due to the lower acidity these vegetables contained having been grown in the Mt. Etna ash soil on Sicily. Va bene!*

* * *

The Basics

Using the cooking method that best matches the ingredients and recipe makes for a successful cooking experience. Cooking methods vary depending on the heat type and moisture used. Food is cooked through the transfer of energy in the form of heat. Heat is transferred through conduction, convection, and radiation or a combination of all three. Cooking methods vary depending on the type of heat and moisture required.

- Dry-heat techniques are often listed as broil, roast, bake, griddle, grill, pan-broil; no liquid or moisture is used when cooking with these methods.

- Dry-heat using fat does not add moisture, but does add fat to preparation such as when you pan-fry, sauté, stir fry, or deep-fry.

- Moist-heat methods will include liquid in cooking, in one way or another such as when you poach, boil, simmer, steam, braise.

Microwave cooking works well for foods containing moisture and is a lifesaver for defrosting or reheating prepared foods. In this method of cooking energy penetrates the food and quickly cooks it.[1]

As you proceed with your culinary experience know that nutrition and flavor go hand in hand. Keep the following tips in mind as you select and prepare ingredients:

- Start with high-quality, fresh ingredients.
- Store food properly until ready for use.
- Use cooking techniques that retain texture, flavor, nutritional value, and color.
- Clean vegetables and fruits well before use.
- Use as little water as possible when cooking produce to retain nutrients. Steam whenever possible.

- Cover most vegetables with a lid during cooking to retain nutrients.

- Save the cooking water from vegetables to use in sauces, soups and stews. This recycles the nutrient-rich liquid back into your body versus ditching it down the drain or in the garbage.

- Try recipes that call for baking, broiling or steaming to help decrease the fat in finished products.

- Meat, fish, and poultry naturally contain fat and some moisture. Keep in mind that as the fat content in meat, fish and poultry decreases the preparation method should include some type of additional moisture to keep the food from drying out.

Be sure to have the right amount of ingredients, the correct equipment, and the time to prepare a recipe from start to finish. Being in a hurry will not speed up the cooking time of a recipe. Nor will cooking something at a temperature higher than called for in hopes that is will get done faster. As your technique improves so will your confidence.

It is critical to have appropriate storage for the food you prepare until it is ready to use or serve. The importance of having access to both a refrigerator and a freezer during your cooking adventures is discussed in the food safety section at the end of this chapter.

The Planning

The military adage *prior planning prevents poor performance* can be applied to meal and menu planning. A menu is simply the various foods offered together that make up a meal. Smart menu planning will save you money, time and extra trips to the grocery store to buy items you forgot. Variety is important to successful menu planning. Include foods from all food groups that vary in texture, flavor, temperature, and color. Choose foods that are nutrient dense instead of just loaded with calories. Apply your nutrition knowledge to make healthy food choices. Good menu planning considers the cost, food preparation time, likes and dislikes, and the activities and schedules of those who will be eating from your menu.[2] Finally, balance higher cost foods with lower cost foods so your menu fits within your budget.

The List

Once you've chosen a recipe to prepare check your cupboards, refrigerator and freezer for the ingredients needed and add them to your grocery list. Add to your list:

- Foods to round out the rest of the menu that includes your recipe

- Foods you're running low on

- Foods on your menu for the next week of meals plus healthy snacks

- General amounts you need next to each item

Appendix D contains a healthy eating shopping list to help you get started.

The Shopping Strategies

With your grocery list in hand let's go grocery shopping. First, select a couple stores close by with the best overall quality of foods and best prices. Then adopt these strategies to make your trip a success.

- *Eat before you shop.* Shopping on an empty stomach will only entice you to buy foods you wouldn't otherwise buy if your stomach was full.

- Wear comfortable shoes for walking the aisles and a sweater or jacket in case the inside of store is cold. Far too many of my shopping trips have been cut short because the store was too cold.

- Use reusable shopping bags. Don't have any? Alternatives are to reuse the bags you received from a previous grocery shopping trip. Do your part to be *green* helping to save the environment. Leave the extra space in the trashcan for unavoidable waste. For good sanitation, wash your reusable bags periodically.

- Purchase items in boxes rather than the six-pack plastic ring holders. Birds or other animals have been known to get their head caught in the ring once the rings are dumped at the local landfill. If you must buy food in such holders, cut the rings apart with a scissors or knife before tossing in the recycle bin.

- Read the label to set a healthy table. Use Appendix A as a guide to easy food label reading and comparison shopping to get the most nutrition and best deal.

- *Shop the perimeter of the grocery store.* The more healthy foods such as dairy, meats, breads and produce line the outside aisles of the store.

- Center aisles of the supermarket offer mostly prepared foods— many high in fat and calories. The basic categories of food to shop for are fruits and vegetables, bread and cereals, milk and dairy products, meat, poultry, fish and beans, and seasonings such as herbs, spices, oil and vinegar, fats and sweets.

Shopping Aisle by Aisle

The goal when grocery shopping is to make as many healthy food choices as possible often. I designed this guide to help you shop with good health and a frugal budget in mind. Coupled with the healthy eating shopping list you create or the one from Appendix D your shopping trip will be a success. *Yes it will!*

Grains: whole grain, high fiber—a good deal

- By far breads, cereals, pastas, and other grain product can contribute the most meal for your money. Choose breads and cereals that have the words *100% whole grain* on the label, contain at least *three grams of fiber and less than five grams of sugar* per serving.

- Go for whole-grain cooked and ready-to-eat cereals like oatmeal and Shredded Wheat™ or store brand equal. Be aware that instant or quick cooking hot or ready-to-eat cereals are usually higher in sodium and or sugar. Sodium and sugar make these cereals appealing to children and those accustomed to a high sodium, high sugar diet while serving as preservatives and speeding up cooking time. Whole grain foods are more nutritious than refined grains since they have more fiber and are more filling. Choose brown or wild rice, buckwheat, popcorn, barley, bulgur, whole wheat couscous, whole grain cornmeal, bread or crackers, whole wheat tortillas and whole grain pasta and noodles.

- Regular white rice and brown rice will generally cost less than rice that is instant, seasoned, precooked, or quick-cooking.

- Don't forget the day old bread section where you can purchase baked items for a bargain price. Bakery outlet stores also offer wholesome breads and cereals at significantly reduced prices.

Dairy: milk, yogurt, cheese and milk alternatives

- Less fat generally means lower cost.

- Choose fat-free and low-fat dairy products. Whole milk products often cost more and nutritionally mean more heart clogging saturated fat. *All milk is an excellent source of calcium.* Fat, not calcium, is removed in low-fat or nonfat milk. Drink up.

- Buying in bulk or larger containers will often translate into cheaper prices per serving. Be sure you will use it all before it outdates or it's not a bargain.

Protein Foods:

- For beef pick lean cuts that have *loin or round* in their name. *Choice and Select* cuts are lower in fat than prime cuts and provide the most servings per pound.

- Chicken, ground beef, pork shoulder, turkey, and beef liver can be some of your best buys at the market. Select ground beef that is 90% lean or greater.

- Lower cost cuts of meats can be just as nutritious per serving as higher cost cuts of meat. Make the fattier cuts of meat an occasional choice, once a month or less, not an everyday habit. Select leaner cuts of meat and poultry using these examples:
  Beef: Eye of round, top round steak, top sirloin, and chuck roast
  Lamb: Leg of lamb, arm chop and loin chop
  Pork: Center loin chop or roast, lean ham, sirloin chops, top loin
  Poultry: Select white meat chicken and turkey. Remove the visible fat before cooking and remove the skin before eating. The white meat from the breast of poultry contains less fat than the dark meat. Select ground breast meat of chicken and turkey for lower fat options.[3]

- Luncheon meat: Choose lean beef, turkey, ham, or low fat luncheon meats for sandwiches instead of higher fat options like salami and regular bologna.[3] Apply the once or less a month rule for the fattier luncheon meat choices.

- Excellent and more economical sources of protein include dried peas and beans, eggs, and peanut butter. Both dried beans and peas are excellent sources of fiber and low in fat. Cheese is usually named as part of the dairy group, but it is also a meat alternate, providing about seven grams of protein per ounce. Be careful though as that one ounce of cheese can contain more than double the calories and fat ounce per ounce as the leanest beef or chicken breast.

Fruits and vegetables: canned, frozen or fresh—a matter of taste and convenience

- Purchase specific types of produce when it's in season for the best deal, best flavor and optimal taste. Table 10.1 below provides a handy list of various types of fruits and vegetables and when they are in season at the grocers or local farmer's market.

Table 10.1 In-season Vegetables and Fruits

WINTER	SPRING	SUMMER	FALL
Avocados	Apricots	Berries	Apples
Broccoli	Artichokes	Beets	Beets
Brussels sprouts	Asparagus	Corn	Cauliflower
Cabbage	Berries	Cherries	Cranberries
Cauliflower	Chile peppers	Green beans	Figs
Chinese	Collards	Mangoes	Grapes
cabbage	Mustard greens	Melons	Persimmons
Grapefruit	Peas	Peaches	Pumpkin
Kale	Spinach	Plums	Spinach
Oranges	Strawberries	Summer squash	Rutabagas
Pears	Sweet peppers	Sweet peppers	
Sweet potatoes		Watermelon	
Tangerines			
Winter squash			

Source: Baker S, Sutherland B, Mitchell R, Rogers K. Eating Smart—Being Active. Fort Collins, CO: Colorado State University Extension; 2007.

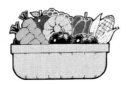

- Research has shown there are only slight nutrient variations between canned, frozen, and fresh vegetables. Comparing the vitamin C content between three forms of a given vegetable you will find the difference is minimal.

- Canned and frozen fruits and vegetables are harvested at their peak, when maximum nutrient levels have been reached and packed and or processed immediately. Since most canned foods are canned raw and cooked in the can there is a small loss of nutrients when canned vegetables are heat processed. Save the liquid from canned fruits and vegetables to use in soups and sauces as an added nutritional and flavor boost to both.

- Strive daily to eat five to nine servings of produce. Research has proven eating a diet rich in fruits and vegetables promotes good health by boosting immunity and reducing the risk of some cancers, high blood pressure, stroke, and diabetes.

- Get in the habit of eating produce often to expand your produce palate. Buy the kinds of produce you're likely to eat and choose to include one new kind of produce you've not tried before each month to expand your produce possibilities.[4,5]

Fats: solid or liquid—the form doesn't change the calorie content

When purchasing oils and hard fats for cooking and general consumption balance quantity, quality, and nutritional benefits. *Refer to the chart in Chapter 5 for suggestions for healthy oils and table fats. Use this chart to help you choose foods with healthier fats when you shop.

Foods with MONO-UNSATURATED FATS (HEALTHY)	Foods with POLY-UNSATURATED FATS (HEALTHY)	Foods with SATURATED FATS (LEAST HEALTHY)
Olives	Corn oil	Butter **
Peanuts	Margarine, tub-type*	Cheese**
Peanut butter	Sunflower seeds	Cream**
Almonds	Flaxseeds	Sour cream**
Almond butter	Walnuts	Half & Half**
Avocados	Sesame seeds	Bacon **
	Tahini	Stick Margarine
	Fatty fish**—salmon, mackerel, trout, sardines	Coconut
		Fatty meat**
		Lunch meat**

*made with PUFA (polyunsaturated fatty acids), **contains cholesterol

- Make monounsaturated and polyunsaturated fats your primary source of dietary fat. This helps prevent chronic diseases by decreasing saturated fat intake.

- For a mild flavored, light colored fat choose canola, corn, safflower, light olive oil, sunflower oil or a combination of these.

- For the best flavor of olive oil use an *extra virgin* variety.

- Butter is a favorite fat that should be consumed in moderation. Small amounts, used judiciously can enhance flavor.

- Choose butter over hydrogenated or stick margarine and shortening that contain *trans* fats.

- Use fat-free butter flavored spray-on fat for coating baking sheets or saucepans to prevent sticking to cookware and eliminate extra calories.

- Typically, fat is 120 calories per tablespoon regardless of its physical form.

- If you are unsure about the fat in a food you are buying, read the Nutrition Facts Label for saturated fat and trans fat amounts.

● ● ●

OIL TIP: *The three enemies of oils are: oxygen, sunlight and heat. Store oils in a dark, cool place with the lid tightened down snuggly.*

● ● ●

Miscelleous: Sweets, snack foods, and alcoholic beverages

- Sweets, snack foods, and alcoholic beverages can quickly run up your grocery bill and calorie intake without providing much nutrition.

- Purchase items from this category at discount stores to save money and consume in moderation if at all.

The Freezer

Eating frozen and pre-prepared foods, especially many types of produce, can be just as healthy as eating fresh. The kinds of foods I'm referring to here are foods frozen without added processing and sauces. Both nutritionally and economically, frozen foods have advantages over fresh by saving both time and money. Follow these basic frozen food principles listed below and you will be ahead economically and nutritionally.

- Choose frozen foods without obvious ice crystals. Ice crystals may indicate the food has been thawed and refrozen, reducing quality, but may be still safe to eat. When in doubt, pass it by.

- Once you get food home, label the packages with the date of purchase. Most frozen food should be used within one to six months of purchase or by the *use by date* on the label.

- Use food frozen the longest time, first.

- When thawing frozen foods, only thaw the amount you are going to use. For food safety reasons never place completely thawed foods back into the freezer.[6]

Consider including frozen vegetables, frozen fruits, frozen chicken, fish and meat on your menu to save time and money. Add a fresh salad and a tall glass of nonfat milk for a complete and nutritionally balanced meal.

Trim—Skim—Chill

Your shopping trip has been a success and now you are ready to prepare the first of many delicious and healthy meals. To assure that you do not go from healthy to hazardous to your health, practice these basic and simple culinary methods to cut back on the fat in the foods you prepare:

- Remove visible fat on poultry and meat before cooking.

- Roast, bake, broil, grill or boil poultry or beef versus frying.

- Skim off all visible fat that rises to the top of soups or stews by dragging a lettuce leaf through the top of the mixture; the fat will adhere to the leaf. Then discard the leaf.

- Chill soups or stews containing cooked meat or poultry then skim off the fat that rises to the top.

- Cook and crumble ground beef, drain in a colander, then rinse with very hot water and drain well.

- Avoid using fat laden sauces and dressings on vegetables, salads, or meats.

The Safety

Food safety and sanitation are top priorities anytime food is stored or served. Remember this food safety motto: *when in doubt throw it out.* Never take chances where food safety is involved. You can't taste botulism or other food bacteria and toxins. *Never* taste potentially harmful food to see if it's still good or not spoiled. That is nonsense and can be deadly. You are worth more than the opened $3.00 jar of mayonnaise you accidentally left out on the counter overnight.

The best reference for all aspects of food safety from food selection and preparation to service and storage is free online from the USDA titled: *Kitchen Companion: Your Safe Food Handbook.* For your own copy go to the link: http://www.fsis.usda.gov/PDF/Kitchen_Companion.pdf or request a copy via the mail using the contacts listed in the *resource section* under *food safety, labeling and advertising.* It covers the *clean, separate, cook and chill* guidelines of food safety:

- Clean hands, food contact surfaces, and vegetables and fruits.

- Separate raw, cooked, and ready-to-eat foods while shopping, storing, and preparing foods.

- Cook foods to a safe temperature.

- Chill (refrigerate) perishable foods promptly.[6]

Keeping food safe begins with good hygiene. Wash your hands with warm water and soap thoroughly and rinse with warm water often before, during, and after food preparation. Handwashing is the number one defense against foodborne illness and deters the everyday flu or cold bug. How long should you wash your hands? A good rule of thumb is to slowly sing the tune Happy Birthday repeating it while you lather up, about 20 seconds. Dry with a clean, dry towel dedicated for only this purpose. A single use, disposable towel is preferable. Have a cut or sore on your hands? Wear disposable gloves to avoid the spread of germs. Always avoid sneezing or coughing over food.

Use a separate cutting board for raw meat, fish, poultry or egg products to avoid cross-contamination with cooked foods of these types. *Never* place cooked, uncovered foods on surfaces exposed to raw foods—plates, counters, cutting boards or mats, or any other surface without first cleaning the surfaces with hot, soapy water, and then rinsing with hot water. Let the surface air dry.

And I repeat, you should have access to a refrigerator and a freezer during your cooking adventures. Perishable foods like raw eggs, poultry, meat, and seafood must be properly refrigerated. The internal temperature of the refrigerator should be 33°F to 40°F. The internal temperature of the freezer should be -20°F to 0°F.

The coldest part of the refrigerator or freezer box is located at the back of the box. For safe storage of foods that spoil easily if exposed to warmer temperatures stow these items in the back of the box. Less temperature sensitive foods such as juice, uncut produce, and starchy low protein foods can be stored more near the front, and condiments like ketchup, mustard, and pickles in the refrigerator door.

Harmful bacteria are destroyed when foods are cooked thoroughly to the recommended internal temperature before eating. Proper temperature for doneness depends on the food type and its protein content. Don't guess. Use a food thermometer to check for doneness. Table 10.1 lists the safe minimum internal temperature chart for various vulnerable foods.

Table 10.2 Safe Minimum Internal Food Temperatures

Foods	Temperature in °F
Ground Meat & Meat Mixtures	
Beef, Pork, Veal, Lamb	160
Turkey, Chicken	165
Fresh Beef, Veal, Lamb	
Steaks, roasts, chops	145
Poultry	
Chicken & turkey, whole	165
Poultry breasts, roasts	165
Poultry thighs, legs, wings	165
Duck & goose	165
Stuffing (cooked alone or in bird)	165
Fresh Pork	
Ham	160
Precooked (to reheat)	140
Fresh (raw)	160
Eggs & Egg Dishes	
Eggs: Cook until yolk and white are firm	160
Egg dishes	160
Leftovers & Casseroles	165

Source: USDA, Food Safety and Inspection Service. Available at: http://www.fsis.usda.gov/PDF/ Kitchen_Companion.pdf. Accessed February 13, 2011.

Never eat raw eggs (This includes licking the cake batter bowl or eating the cookie dough—sorry!). Raw eggs may contain harmful bacteria that are easily killed during cooking. Always keep eggs stored in their original carton, in the coldest part of the refrigerator. *Never* store eggs, raw or cooked, at room temperature for more than two hours. Eggs are not granted eternal shelf life once they are hard cooked. Hard cooked eggs can be safely stored at refrigerator temperature for up to a total of seven days.

Just like it is not wise to thaw meat, fish, or poultry on the countertop at room temperature, it is a bad food safety practice to leave cooked leftovers out to cool before refrigerating. This practice was common in days when refrigerators were much less efficient and foods would warm up the interior of the refrigerator. If in doubt, place leftovers in a shallow container and set in a pan large enough to hold ice and the leftovers container. Then refrigerate or freeze as appropriate.[6]

* * *

FIRE FIRE FIRE: *Every kitchen, no matter how large or small, should be equipped with a fire extinguisher. Contact your local fire department on the best kind to buy and how to use and maintain it for optimal results. Besides being heroic public servants, firefighters are typically pretty good cooks.*

* * *

Now let's start cookin'!

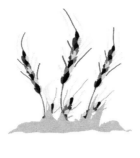

ELEVEN

EZ RECIPES: A TO Z

Nutrition doesn't start until the food passes the lips.

In the midst of the completion of this book my beloved Maltese, Toni Lee nearly 17 years old went to Heaven. I'm told the furniture in Heaven is made of liver treats. In the final months of her life, Toni patiently supervised my kitchen testing all 26 recipes in this chapter. Which was her favorite recipe? Beer Butt Chicken, of course.

Getting Started

Are you too busy to cook? I understand your plight. Cook anyway. Cooks are cool people. Be cool. Included in this *cookbook-in-a-book* are 26 recipes, one for every letter of the alphabet each with a story or tip, a cooking equipment list, ingredients, instructions, and nutritional analysis.

The recipes range from simple to challenging. After having prepared and eaten food from each recipe I am pleased to report this chapter tastes the best. I hope you'll enjoy the outcome of each recipe you test. A few years ago God arranged for me to move into a neighborhood with great cooks who have since willingly sampled these recipes with excellent reviews. *Bon Appétit.*

A   **A+ Honor Rolls**
B   **Best Banana Bread**
C   **Beer Butt Chicken**
D   **Delicious Summer Salad**
E   **Deviled Eggs**
F   **Fresh Sicilian Fennel Salad**
G   **Baked Garlic Spread**
H   **Holiday Hot House Cider**
I   **Drew's Incredible Almond Biscotti**
J   **Jumpin' Jack Banana Pancakes**
K   **Kiwi & Strawberry Salad**
L   **Liver & Onions**
M   **Perfect Mashed Potatoes**
N   **Navy Bean & Ham**
O   **Opal Salad**
P   **Polish Gulumki**
Q   **Quick Baked Wild Salmon**
R   **Kansas State Game Day Pot Roast**
S   **Sicilian Pasta Sauce**
T   **Fresh Tomato and Basil Salad**
U   **Pineapple Coconut Upside Down Cake**
V   **Steamed Vegetables—Broccoli**
W   **Walk the Trail Mix**
X   **X-tra EZ Energy Bars**
Y   **Baked Yams**
Z   **Reduced Fat Zucchini Bread**

Refer to Appendix E for definitions of culinary terms. Refer to Appendix F for ingredient substitutions. Refer to Appendix G for measurements and conversions of ingredients.

NUTRITION NOTES: A 10-nutrient nutrition analysis was completed on each recipe using the USDA National Nutrient Database for Standard Reference, Release 23. This reference is the baseline for most food and nutrition databases in the US, and is used in food policy, research, and nutrition monitoring. Abbreviations include carbohydrates (Carbs), cholesterol (Chol), grams (g), and milligrams (mg). No ingredients with trans fats were used in the production of these recipes. The analysis is an estimate of the quantities of nutrients found in each recipe. If you have a medical condition that recommends you avoid specific nutrients or foods, consult a registered dietitian for additional guidance.

The Potato Experiment

If you're new to the kitchen begin your culinary journey with mastering the art of baking a potato. Don't worry, you have plenty of time. You won't bake the potato, your oven will. In less time than it takes to sit through a traffic light changing from red to green in Fort Worth, Texas you'll have a potato baking in the oven.

Preheat the oven at 375°F. Wash the potato under cool, running water and pierce it with a fork to make a place for the steam to escape as it cooks. Place the potato in the oven for 45 minutes. The potato is done and ready to eat when it gives to gentle pressure. Is that it? That's it.

A is for A+ Honor Rolls

Yield: 24 rolls

This is a great tasting basic bread roll recipe. Be patient, read the directions through completely and allow plenty of time to prepare this recipe. The best way to set the tone for showing a house that's up for sale or rent is to bake some bread. The aroma that bursts into the air will put the prospective buyers at ease. As you wait for the dough to rise turn to Appendix H for more on my love affair with bread.
Source: Adapted from the original recipe by Mary Hotchkiss.

Oven temperature: 375°F or 190°C

Equipment: 2 baking sheets, measuring cups, 3-quart mixing bowl, large cutting board, rolling pin, table knife, oven mitts, oven, cooling rack, pancake turner, kitchen timer

Ingredients:
   1 c lukewarm water (about 90°F)
   1 packet dry yeast
   ½ c granulated sugar
   1 stick salted butter, melted and cooled
   3 large eggs, whole, raw, room temperature
   4½ c + 1/2 c unbleached all purpose flour

Directions:
1. Spray two baking sheets with nonstick cooking spray and set aside.
2. In a large mixing bowl dissolve the yeast in the water.
3. Gently add the sugar, eggs and melted butter to the dissolved yeast, one at a time, combining well.
4. Add 3 cups of the flour to the liquid mixture and beat until smooth.
5. Add the remaining 1½ cups of flour slowly, beating until the dough is easy to handle. The dough will appear slightly sticky to the touch. The dough will rise in the same bowl it was prepared in.
6. Cover the dough with wax paper and a damp towel and let rise in a warm place until double in size, about 1 hour. The dough

is ready when you gently press down on the dough and the indention remains.

7. Generously dust a large cutting board or clean, flat surface with flour.

8. Turn the dough onto the dusted surface and divide into two pieces.

9. Working with one piece at a time, dust the top of the dough and the rolling pin with flour and roll the dough into a 10-inch circle.

10. Cut the circle into 12 pie shaped wedges.

11. Starting with the wider, rounded edge, tightly roll the dough towards the pointed end.

12. Place rolls onto a baking sheet, shaping each into a half-moon shape.

13. Repeat with the remaining half. Place 12 rolls on each baking sheet.

14. Set dough aside in a warm place to rise until nearly double in size, about 1 hour.

15. Preheat oven to 375°. Place one pan of rolls in the oven and bake for 8 to 10 minutes, until golden brown. Remove from the oven and with the pancake turner gently remove the rolls from the baking sheets onto a cooling rack.

16. Repeat the baking process with the second half allowing enough time for the oven to return to 375°F or 190°C before proceeding.

Serve rolls warm or cool completely to room temperature and store in an air tight container.

Serving size: 1 roll

Calories	Fiber (g)	Carbs (g)	Protein (g)	Fat (g)
155	1 g	24 g	4 g	5 g
Chol (mg)	Sodium (mg)	Iron (mg)	Calcium (mg)	Potassium (mg)
33 mg	43 mg	1 mg	9 mg	41 mg

B is for Best Banana Bread

Yield: 1 loaf or 16 slices

Over ripe bananas make the best banana bread. Try this easy and delicious quick bread recipe that requires little preparation. Served still warm, banana bread is great with coffee.
Source: Adapted from the original recipe by Evelyn Shaw.

Oven temperature: 350°F or 177°C

Equipment: oven, measuring cups, measuring spoons, 3-quart mixing bowl, electric hand mixer, 1 loaf pan, oven mitts, serrated knife, cooling rack, timer

Ingredients:

½ c canola oil

2 eggs, medium, whole, raw

2 c unbleached all purpose flour, sifted

¼ c black walnuts, chopped

1 T vanilla extract

1 c brown sugar, packed

1 t baking soda

3 bananas, medium, ripened

Instructions:

Preheat oven to 350°F. Spray an 8½" x 4½" x 2½" loaf pan with nonstick cooking spray and set aside.

1. Mash the bananas until smooth and set aside.

2. Combine baking soda and flour in a separate bowl.

3. Beat eggs for 30 seconds.

4. Add the oil, sugar, and eggs stirring until creamy.

5. Blend bananas into mixture until smooth.

6. Stir in flour and baking soda until just moistened.

7. Add nuts and vanilla extract.

8. Beat for 30 seconds at medium speed with hand mixer.

9. Pour mixture into the prepared pan.

Bake for 55 to 65 minutes or until a wooden toothpick inserted in the center of the loaf comes out clean. Remove loaf from the oven and leave in pan to cool for 10 minutes. Gently loosen the loaf from the sides of the pan with a knife and remove loaf from pan. Let the bread cool completely on a wire cooling rack. Using a serrated knife, cut into ½ inch slices.

Serving size: 1 slice

Calories	Fiber (g)	Carbs (g)	Protein (g)	Fat (g)
211	1	31	3	9
Chol (mg)	**Sodium (mg)**	**Iron (mg)**	**Calcium (mg)**	**Potassium (mg)**
20	91	1	19	133

C is for Beer Butt Chicken

Yield: 8 pieces

You must try this recipe. Baking a whole chicken propped up by a half-full can of beer and on its own legs is a unique cooking experience.

Oven temperature: 375°F or 190°C

Equipment: oven, beer can, foil, baking sheet, disposable gloves, oven mitts, timer, measuring spoons, measuring cups, 1-quart mixing bowl, meat thermometer

Ingredients:
    2 6-inch sprigs of fresh rosemary
    non-stick cooking spray
    3 T parsley, dried
    2 t paprika
    3 T garlic powder
    ¼ t sea salt
    ¼ t pepper, ground
    3 lbs chicken, whole
    12 oz beer, light, with can

Instructions:

Remove all but one oven rack from the oven and move the remaining rack to the lowest position in the oven. Preheat the oven to 375°F. Cover baking sheet with foil and set aside.

Before opening, clean the outside of the beer can with soapy water and rinse well with hot water and dry outside of can. Open the can and pour out 6 ounces of the beer.

1. In a bowl mix together parsley, paprika, garlic powder, salt and pepper as the seasoning rub for the outside of the bird.

2. Put on disposable gloves before handling the bird.

3. Remove and dispose of the liver, gizzard, and or neck that may be in the cavity of the bird.

4. Insert the rosemary sprigs deep inside the bird.

5. Place the chicken over the open end of the upright beer can, insert the can into the cavity of the bird using the can and the legs of the chicken to hold the bird upright.

6. Place the bird on the baking sheet.

7. Spray the outside of the bird with non-stick cooking spray and generously cover it seasoning rub.

8. Dispose of the gloves.

9. Roast beer butt chicken to an internal temperature of 165°F or 74°C for about 80 minutes. Test for doneness in the most dense (thickest) area of the breast, using an instant read or meat thermometer. Serve hot.

Serving size: 1/8 chicken

Calories	Fiber (g)	Carbs (g)	Protein (g)	Fat (g)
203	< 1	4	20	11
Chol (mg)	Sodium (mg)	Iron (mg)	Calcium (mg)	Potassium (mg)
60	136	2	24	251

D is for Delicious Summer Salad

Yield: 10 cups

This robust and colorful salad is rich in flavor and phytonutrients. Clean produce well under cool, running water before preparation. Dab leafy greens with a clean, dry towel to remove excess water.

Equipment: cutting board, sharp knife, large salad bowl, measuring cup, measuring spoons, clean dry towel, 1 cup container with lid

Ingredients:

4 c spinach, fresh

1 c arugula, torn into bite-size pieces

4 c lettuce, green leaf, torn into bite-size pieces

½ c radishes, red, raw, sliced into thin slices

½ c broccoli florets, fresh, torn into bite-size pieces

½ c carrots, cut into coin-sized pieces

1 c cherry tomatoes, raw, halved

1 medium cucumber, raw, with peel, cut into coin-sized pieces

¼ c onion, green/spring, raw, chopped

1 T olive oil, extra-virgin

1 T balsamic vinegar

¼ t sea salt

¼ t pepper, freshly ground

Instructions:

1. Gently toss the vegetable together in a large bowl and set aside at room temperature for 20 minutes. If prepared ahead of time, cover and refrigerate until 20 minutes before serving.

2. In a 1 cup container combine the vinegar, salt and pepper; cover with the lid and shake vigorously.

3. Drizzle over salad and gently toss. Serve immediately.

Serving size: 1 cup

Calories	Fiber (g)	Carbs (g)	Protein (g)	Fat (g)
47	1	4	1	2
Chol (mg)	**Sodium (mg)**	**Iron (mg)**	**Calcium (mg)**	**Potassium (mg)**
0	82	7	4	239

E is for Deviled Eggs

Yield: 24 halves

This recipe is a family favorite. Eggs are an inexpensive source of protein. Egg shells contain calcium and will fortify your compost for later recycling into your garden soil. Make sure that you rinse the shells well before adding to the compost to remove any protein left from the egg white.
Source: Patty Gallagher

Equipment: 2-quart saucepan with lid, measuring cups, measuring spoons, tablespoon, sharp knife, 1-quart mixing bowl, fork, teaspoon

Ingredients:

12 eggs, chicken, whole, medium, raw

1½ quarts cold water

4 T mayonnaise

¼ t paprika

Instructions:

1. Fill a 2-quart saucepan with cold water and add eggs. On high heat, bring eggs to a boil. Once at a steady boil turn off heat immediately and cover with the lid. Leave covered on range for 15 minutes.

2. Pour off water and bathe eggs in cold water. Carefully peel eggs under cool running water. To peel, gently tap the egg on a hard surface until it cracks and remove all of the shell.

3. Cool eggs in the refrigerator for 15-20 minutes. Cut each egg into halves lengthwise and scoop out yolk. Set aside egg whites in the refrigerator.

4. Mash yolks then add mayonnaise to the yolks stirring until smooth.

5. Spoon a teaspoon of the mixture into the empty yoke cavity, filling to just above the white. Arrange on a serving plate and lightly sprinkle with paprika. Cover.

Keep refrigerated until ready to serve. Serve chilled.

Serving size: 1 half

Calories	Fiber (g)	Carbs (g)	Protein (g)	Fat (g)
55	0	0	3	5
Chol (mg)	**Sodium (mg)**	**Iron (mg)**	**Calcium (mg)**	**Potassium (mg)**
94	44	0	13	32

F is for Fresh Sicilian Fennel Salad

Yield: 3 cups

This Sicilian summertime salad favorite is made with fennel. Pronounced finocchio in Italian, fennel has a crunchy texture and the mild flavor of licorice. Molto Buono!

Equipment: sharp knife, cutting board, measuring spoons, 3-quart mixing bowl, large spoon

Ingredients:
   1 fennel bulb, large (about 8 oz)
   ½ onion, large (about 3 oz)
   7 fresh basil leaves
   1 t balsamic vinegar
   1 T olive oil, extra-virgin
   1/8 t sea salt

Instructions:

1.   Clean the vegetables well under cool, running water before preparation. Dab with a clean, dry towel to remove excess water. Trim the tough upper branches from fennel bulb.

2.   Cut the fennel and onion in half lengthwise, and then slice crosswise into thin pieces.

3.   Roll-up the basil leaves one at a time and cut into thin strips crosswise.

4.   Combine all the ingredients into one bowl and gently toss until well blended. Let rest for 20 minutes at room temperature. If made ahead, cover and refrigerate until 20 minutes before service. Serve immediately.

Serving size: ¾ cup

Calories	Fiber (g)	Carbs (g)	Protein (g)	Fat (g)
57	2	6	1	4
Chol (mg)	**Sodium (mg)**	**Iron (mg)**	**Calcium (mg)**	**Potassium (mg)**
0	104	1	35	274

G is for Baked Garlic Spread

Yield: 40 cloves

This easy recipe is a healthy party favorite for any occasion.

Oven temperature: 400°F or 205°C

Equipment: oven, muffin tin, foil, sharp knife, measuring spoons, oven mitts

Ingredients:

4 garlic bulbs

4 T olive oil, extra-virgin

Instructions:

Preheat oven to 400°F.

1. From the non-root end of each garlic bulb, cut horizontally enough of the dried peel and meat to see the fleshy fresh insides. Place each bulb cut-side up in separate muffin tin wells.

2. Drizzle 1 tablespoon of the oil over each bulb getting as much between the clove spaces as possible. Cover bulbs with foil folding the edges under the tin to make a tight seal.

3. Bake for 15 minutes. Remove the foil and continue to bake uncovered until cloves are soft to the touch, about 15 minutes longer. Serve warm with sourdough bread or crackers.

Serving size: 2 cloves

Calories	Fiber (g)	Carbs (g)	Protein (g)	Fat (g)
32	0	2	0	3
Chol (mg)	**Sodium (mg)**	**Iron (mg)**	**Calcium (mg)**	**Potassium (mg)**
0	1	0	11	24

H is for Holiday Hot House Cider

Yield: 8 cups

This non-alcoholic holiday cider is tasty and nutritious. Stir the mixture before serving to keep the ground cinnamon from clumping.

Equipment: 5-quart non-reactive pot or Dutch oven, measuring cups, measuring spoons, range, large spoon (a slow cooker would work well for this)

Ingredients:

½ gallon apple juice, 100% juice

6 cloves

1 t ground cinnamon or 2 cinnamon stick

1 t (about 20 seeds) whole allspice

Instructions:

1. Combine all the ingredients in a large pot and simmer on low heat for about 30 minutes.

2. Stir frequently.

3. Serve hot, 180°F or 82°C.

Serving size: 1 cup

Calories	Fiber (g)	Carbs (g)	Protein (g)	Fat (g)
116	< 1	29	0	0
Chol (mg)	Sodium (mg)	Iron (mg)	Calcium (mg)	Potassium (mg)
0	10	0	25	255

I is for Drew's Incredible Almond Biscotti

Yield: 40 biscotti

Biscotti, in Italian, means twice baked cookie, is great dunked in and eaten with a tall glass of fat-free milk. Be patient with this advanced recipe, read the directions thoroughly, and allow plenty of time to prepare it.
Source: Jennifer Moran

Oven temperature: 350°F or 177°C

Equipment: measuring cups, measuring spoons, sharp knife, cutting board, oven mitts, 2 baking sheets, cooling racks, wooden toothpicks, 12 inch ruler

Ingredients:

3½ c + ½ c unbleached all purpose flour

1½ t baking powder

4½ t anise seed

1½ c almonds, whole, raw

3 eggs, whole, large, raw

1¼ c sugar, granulated

¼ t salt

1½ t vanilla extract

½ c butter, melted and cooled

Instructions:

Preheat oven to 350°F. Spray two baking sheets with nonstick cooking spray and set aside.

1.   Coarsely chop ½ cup of the almonds with a sharp knife. Set aside.

2.   In a large bowl combine 3½ c flour, baking powder, anise, and all the almonds. Set aside.

3.   In a separate bowl combine the eggs, salt, and vanilla. Beat mixture with a mixer on high speed for 4 to 5 minutes or until thoroughly combined.

4.   Add the sugar ¼ cup at a time until the mixture has a light yellow foamy appearance and when poured from a spoon looks like a yellow ribbon.

5.   Add wet mixture to the dry ingredients and stir together until thoroughly combined.

6.   Lightly dust a large cutting board or clean, flat surface with flour.

7.   Turn half of the mixture onto the dusted surface and form one 10x4 inch log. Dough may be sticky; wet hands with cool water to handle dough more easily. Repeat with the remaining half. Pat down each loaf to make it 1 inch tall. Place each loaf in the center of a prepared baking sheet.

8.   Bake each loaf until it is firm to the touch not giving to gentle pressure, about 20 to 25 minutes.

9.   Rotate sheets halfway through the baking cycle for even browning. Test for doneness by inserting a wooden toothpick into the center of a loaf; it is done if it comes out clean.

10. Remove loaves from the oven and let cool for about 10 minutes.

11. Reduce oven temperature to 300°F.

12. Once each loaf is cool enough to handle, using a sharp knife, cut straight down, crosswise, through each loaf, into ½ inch slices.

13. Lay each slice on its side on baking sheets a single layer.

14. Return baking sheets to the oven and bake biscotti until slices are lightly golden on each side, about 7 to 10 minutes per side, turning slices over once during this baking cycle.

15. Remove from the oven and transfer the biscotti from the baking sheets to cooling racks. Biscotti will become crisp as it cools.

Serve immediately or store in air tight containers.

Serving size: 1 biscotti

Calories	Fiber (g)	Carbs (g)	Protein (g)	Fat (g)
128	1	17	3	6
Chol (mg)	**Sodium (mg)**	**Iron (mg)**	**Calcium (mg)**	**Potassium (mg)**
20	59	1	31	61

J is for Jumpin' Jack Banana Pancakes

Yield: seven 5-inch pancakes

These eat now or pop in the toaster later whole wheat pancakes can be made with blueberries or bananas. The pancakes store easily in plastic storage bags in the refrigerator for up to 5 days.
Source: Jennifer Moran

Equipment: two 1-quart mixing bowls, measuring cups and spoons, wire whisk, pancake turner, 9-inch skillet, 1-quart freezer storage bags

Ingredients:

1¼ c whole wheat flour

2 T brown sugar, packed

3 T flax seed, ground

2 t baking powder

1 1/3 c non-fat milk

2 T canola oil

1 T vanilla

2 bananas, medium, ripe

non-stick cooking spray

Instructions:

1. In a mixing bowl combine dry ingredients.

2. Thoroughly combine wet ingredients in a separate bowl.

3. Add to the dry ingredients stirring well with a wire whisk.

4. Wash the outside of the bananas and peel. Cut the fruit first lengthwise and then crosswise. Fold the fruit pieces into the batter.

5.   Spray a non-stick 9-inch skillet lightly with non-stick cooking spray and place on medium heat until the spray beads up.

6.   Pour ½ cup of batter into the center of the hot skillet. Cook until the outsides of the pancake are opaque, its center just starts to bubble and the bottom is golden brown.

7.   Slide the pancake turner under the center of the pancake and turn it over in one gentle motion to cook the other side until golden brown.

8.   Remove skillet from heat and spray with non-stick spray repeating cooking process for each pancake. Serve hot.

Serving Size: 1 pancake

Calories	Fiber (g)	Carbs (g)	Protein (g)	Fat (g)
191	4	31	5	6
Chol (mg)	Sodium (mg)	Iron (mg)	Calcium (mg)	Potassium (mg)
2	162	1	154	304

K is for Kiwi & Strawberry Salad

Yield: 2 quarts

This easy to prepare salad recipe is loaded with phytonutrients.

Equipment: clean dish towel, cutting board, sharp knife, measuring cups and spoons, 3-quart mixing bowl, tablespoon

Ingredients:
 ¾ lb kiwi (3-4 fruits)
 1 lb strawberries
 3 mint leaves
 ½ c ginger ale
 1 t honey

Instructions:

1. In cool water wash the fruit and mint. Dab dry with a clean towel.

2. Peel kiwis and remove stems from strawberries.

3. Cut kiwis into 1/8-inch slices, cutting through the belly of the fruit to make coin-shaped slices then cut again crosswise.

4. Cut strawberries lengthwise into 1/8-inch slices. Roll-up mint leaves and coarsely chop.

5. In a bowl gently combine the fruit and mint.

6. In a 1-cup measure add the honey to the ginger ale until dissolved. 7. Pour the liquid over fruit mixture and gently toss.

Cover and refrigerate until time to serve.

Serving size: ½ cup

Calories	Fiber (g)	Carbs (g)	Protein (g)	Fat (g)
52	2	13	1	0
Chol (mg)	**Sodium (mg)**	**Iron (mg)**	**Calcium (mg)**	**Potassium (mg)**
0	3	0	24	221

L is for Liver and Onions

Yield: 5 servings

Liver is an excellent source of essential nutrients including iron. This tender and luscious liver recipe can turn tough if overcooked.

Equipment: sharp knife, cutting board, measuring cups and spoons, small bowl, range, 9-inch diameter skillet with lid, 1-quart saucepan

Ingredients:

½ t black pepper, ground

1/3 c unbleached all purpose flour

1/8 c canola oil

1 lb beef liver, baby calf

½ lb onion, sliced

1 beef bouillon cube or 1 t beef bouillon seasoning

1 c hot water

Instructions:

1. Heat the water to boiling and dissolve the bouillon in the hot water. Set aside.

2. Slice the onion into 1/8-inch thick slices.

3. Combine the pepper and flour in a bowl.

4. Cut the liver into five equal pieces then coat the liver with the flour mixture.

5. Add oil to a 9-inch skillet, heat on medium, and brown the liver on each side until lightly browned or about three to five minutes. Reduce heat to low.

6. In the skillet evenly spread the onions evenly over the liver; pour the bouillon over the liver and onions. Bring liquid to a simmer. Cover the skillet with a lid and cook until well done, about 10 minutes (internal temperature of 160°F). Do not overcook.

Serve hot.

Serving size: 3 ounces (deck of cards sized)

Calories	Fiber (g)	Carbs (g)	Protein (g)	Fat (g)
246	1	15	24	10
Chol (mg)	**Sodium (mg)**	**Iron (mg)**	**Calcium (mg)**	**Potassium (mg)**
324	292	6	18	373

M is for Perfect Mashed Potatoes

Yield: 2 cups

Leave the skins on the potatoes to add fiber to this recipe and save the water the potatoes are cooked in for use in a soup or stew.

Equipment: vegetable brush, sharp knife, 3-quart pot with lid, range, measuring cups and spoons, 3-quart mixing bowl, potato masher or electric hand mixer, rubber food scraper, tablespoon

Ingredients:

4 c water

1/8 t salt

1 lb potatoes, red russet

1/3 c low-fat milk (1%)

1 T butter, salted

¼ c fresh parsley, chopped (about 3 large sprigs)

Instructions:

1. Fill a pot with enough water to cover the potatoes, add the salt.

2. Wash the potatoes in cool water removing dirt and eyes (the indentations or pits in the potato that will sprout if allowed to) but do not peel.

3. Cut the potatoes into large pieces, add to the boiling water and cook until tender, about 18-20 minutes.

4. Measure milk and let stand at room temperature for 10 minutes before adding as directed.

5. Remove pot from the heat and drain off the water.

6. With a handheld potato masher or electric mixer mash the potatoes in the pot or a mixing bowl until smooth.

7. Slowly add the milk a bit at a time to get the desired consistency.

8. Stir in butter until melted. Serve hot sprinkled with parsley.

Serving size: ½ cup

Calories	Fiber (g)	Carbs (g)	Protein (g)	Fat (g)
134	2	24	3	3
Chol (mg)	**Sodium (mg)**	**Iron (mg)**	**Calcium (mg)**	**Potassium (mg)**
9	113	1	37	482

N is for Navy Beans and Ham

Yield: 10 cups

My mother is the best cook in the world. Here's one of her recipes to prove it. For best results respect the refreshing of the beans with fresh water.

Source: Adapted from the original recipe by Regina C. Kobuszewski.

Equipment: strainer, cutting board, sharp knife, measuring cups and spoons, 3-quart bowl, 4-quart pot, Crockpot™-type cooker, large spoon

Ingredients:

  water
  6 c beans, navy, dry beans
  ½ t baking soda
  ¾ lb pork, ham shank, bone-in
  1 c onion, chopped
  1 bay leaf
  ¼ t salt
  ¼ t pepper

Instructions:

1. Carefully check beans for stones, rocks, or other foreign matter.

2. Rinse beans under cool, running water.

3. In a gallon jar or large bowl cover beans with water and soak for 8 hours. Drain off the water.

4. In a large pot combine the beans and baking soda and cover with fresh water.

5. Simmer for about 30 minutes. Drain off liquid.

6.   Place the ham hock in center of a slow cooker. Add the beans, onions, bay leaf, salt and pepper around the hock. Add about 4 cups of water or enough to just cover the beans, gently stir to combine ingredients.

7.   Cover slow cooker with a lid, turn on low heat for 4½ to 5 hours or until the beans are tender. Serve hot.

Serving size: 1 cup

Calories	Fiber (g)	Carbs (g)	Protein (g)	Fat (g)
222	12	30	18	4
Chol (mg)	Sodium (mg)	Iron (mg)	Calcium (mg)	Potassium (mg)
24	397	3	8	570

O is for Opal Salad

Yield: 7 cups

Opal Salad is my family's holiday favorite recipe. The final steps of this recipe should be done just before serving time.
Source: Adapted from the original recipe by Regina C. Kobuszewski.

Equipment: strainer, 2-quart saucepan with lid, measuring cups and spoons, range, set of mixing bowls, refrigeration, sharp knife, cutting board, electric hand mixer, rubber food scraper, large spoon

Ingredients:

3 c fresh cranberries

1 c water

1 c granulated sugar

1 c green or red seedless grapes

½ c English walnuts

1 c Dream Whip™ Whipped Topping Mix (1, 1.3 oz envelope Dream Whip Whipped Topping Mix prepared as directed using ½ c cold non-fat milk and ½ t vanilla)

2 c miniature marshmallows

Instructions:

1. Prepare and refrigerate the Dream Whip™ until ready to use.

2. Under cool, running water wash cranberries removing shriveled berries and debris.

3. Bring water and sugar to a boil in a saucepan. Add the cranberries and return to a boil. Reduce heat and simmer for 10 minutes stirring frequently; remove from heat and refrigerate until cool.

4.   Once cooled, drain excess liquid from the whole cranberries.

5.   Clean and slice the grapes and refrigerate. Drain any excess liquid from the sliced grapes before adding to the final mixture.

6.   Remove foreign debris for the nuts. Coarsely chop and set aside.

7.   Gently combine Dream Whip™, drained grapes, walnuts, and marshmallows.

8.   Add the cranberries, mixing all the ingredients together with as little folding as possible to evenly distribute. Do not over mix.

Cover and refrigerate until ready to serve. Serve cold.

Serving size: ½ cup

Calories	Fiber (g)	Carbs (g)	Protein (g)	Fat (g)
140	1	28	1	3
Chol (mg)	Sodium (mg)	Iron (mg)	Calcium (mg)	Potassium (mg)
0	10	0	18	72

P is for Polish Gulumki

Yield: 8 rolls

This Polish culinary wonder is tasty, economical and nutritious. Reuse the water used at the start of the recipe in the final cooking step.
Source: Regina C. Kobuszewski

Oven temperature: 350°F or 177°C

Equipment: oven, Dutch oven and lid, oven mitts, tongs, cutting board, sharp knife, large mixing bowl, 3-quart pot, measuring cups and spoons

Ingredients:
  1 medium head of green cabbage
  1 c uncooked white rice, medium grain
  1 t salt
  ½ t pepper
  1 lb ground beef (85% lean, 15% fat)
  ½ lb ground pork
  1 large white onion, chopped

Instructions:
  Preheat oven to 350°F.

1. Boil enough water in a deep pot to cover cabbage head.

2. Reduce heat to a simmer.

3. Clean cabbage under cool, running water.

4. Next you will remove 16 leaves from the cabbage head.

5. Remove the core of the cabbage with a sharp knife. Carefully submerge cabbage head into the hot water until, one by one each outer leaf starts to release from the head. Remove the head from the water and remove the leaf. Repeat this process until all the leaves are released from the head. Return all the leaves to the simmering water and cook until limp.

6. Remove the leaves from the hot water, set aside 16 leaves. Each roll requires two leaves. Reserve the cooking water.

7. Place any additional leftover cabbage pieces in the bottom of ovenproof baking dish.

8. Combine ground meats, rice, salt, pepper, and onions. Place one-eighth of this mixture at the base of a reserved cabbage leaf and loosely roll leaf to completely cover the mixture tucking in sides like a burrito. Do not pack the mixture.

9. Lay the filled leaf seam down into the center of another leaf and repeat the rolling action. Repeat to make a total of 8 rolls.

10. Place rolls seam down in the baking dish.

11. Measure reserved cooking water and add enough water to equal 6 cups.

12. Cover rolls with water. Cover with oven proof lid.

13. Bake at 350°F for 1 ¼ to 1 ½ hours or until the rolls reach an internal temperature of 160°F and the rice is soft and moist. Serve hot.

Serving size: 1 roll

Calories	Fiber (g)	Carbs (g)	Protein (g)	Fat (g)
260	1	24	17	10
Chol (mg)	Sodium (mg)	Iron (mg)	Calcium (mg)	Potassium (mg)
54	338	3	33	288

Q is for Quick Baked Wild Salmon

Yield: 8

Quick and easy to prepare this salmon recipe makes an elegant and nutritious entrée in less than 20 minutes.

Oven temperature: 350°F or 177°C

Equipment: oven, sharp knife, baking sheet, measuring spoon, meat thermometer

Ingredients:

¼ t lemon pepper, coarsely ground

1/8 t cayenne pepper

1 t parsley, dried

1½ lbs filet, fresh wild salmon

Instructions:

Preheat oven to 350°F.

1. Cut fish into 8 equal pieces and place on a baking sheet.

2. Combine the seasonings and sprinkle over the fish.

3. Bake at 350°F for 8-10 minutes, internal temperature of 145°F. Serve hot.

Serving size: 3 ounces

Calories	Fiber (g)	Carbs (g)	Protein (g)	Fat (g)
155	0	0	22	7
Chol (mg)	**Sodium (mg)**	**Iron (mg)**	**Calcium (mg)**	**Potassium (mg)**
60	48	1	14	537

R is for Kansas State University Game Day Pot Roast

Yield: 8

Gently simmered, well seasoned bottom and top round beef roasts can be just as tender and succulent as prime cuts when cooked right. Enjoy.
Source: Adapted from the original recipe by USDA.

Equipment: deep skillet with lid, range, measuring cups and spoons, cutting board, sharp knife, 1-quart bowl, meat thermometer

Ingredients:

  1/2 c onion, raw, chopped

  2 T water

  2 lbs beef, bottom round roast, trimmed of visible fat

  2 c hot water

  1 beef bouillon cube

  2 T pineapple juice, 100% juice

  ¼ t allspice

  1/8 t pepper, ground

Instructions:

1. In a deep skillet simmer onions until tender in 2 tablespoons of water.

2. Add beef to skillet; brown on all sides.

3. In a bowl combine beef bouillon cube with hot water; stir until dissolved. Add pineapple juice, allspice, pepper.

4. Pour liquid over roast. Cover with a lid.

5. Gently simmer over low heat until tender, about 2 hours. Roast is done when internal temperature is 145°F. Remove from heat and let rest for 20 minute before cutting. Serve hot.

Serving size: 3 ounces

Calories	Fiber (g)	Carbs (g)	Protein (g)	Fat (g)
176	0	2	23	8
Chol (mg)	**Sodium (mg)**	**Iron (mg)**	**Calcium (mg)**	**Potassium (mg)**
69	170	2	8	204

S is for Sicilian Pasta Sauce

Yield: 3½ cups

Italy is known for great food, especially pasta sauce. Enjoy this easy Sicilian pasta sauce recipe packed with phytonutrients. E magnifico!
Source: Adapted from the original recipe by Mely Pitto.

Equipment: cutting board, sharp knife, can opener, 3-quart saucepan

Ingredients:

3 T olive oil, extra-virgin

1 large onion, chopped

2 cloves garlic, chopped

1 can (14.5 oz) diced tomatoes in tomato juice

1 can (8 oz) tomato sauce

1 can (4 oz) mushrooms, stems & pieces, drained

1/8 t sea salt

7 basil leaves

Instructions:

1. In a 3-quart saucepan over medium heat brown onion and garlic until barely tender, translucent and soft, about two minutes.

2. Add the tomatoes, sauce, and drained mushrooms to the onion and garlic mixture and bring to boil.

3. Reduce heat and simmer over low heat for 15 minutes stirring often.

4. Roll-up the basil leaves one at a time and cut into thin strips crosswise.

5. Add salt and basil to sauce, cook for 5 minutes. Serve hot over pasta.

Serving size: ½ cup

Calories	Fiber (g)	Carbs (g)	Protein (g)	Fat (g)
110	2	11	2	6
Chol (mg)	**Sodium (mg)**	**Iron (mg)**	**Calcium (mg)**	**Potassium (mg)**
0	63	15	24	438

T is for Fresh Tomato and Basil Salad

Yield: 4 cups

This Sicilian summertime salad favorite made with tomatoes, onions and basil is flavorful, aromatic and nutritious. For the most flavor and nutrition, store whole tomatoes at room temperature. Once cut, refrigerate, **only if** *its serving time is over two hours of after the preparation time.*

Equipment: sharp knife, cutting board, measuring spoons, 3-quart mixing bowl, large spoon

Ingredients:
  4 medium tomatoes, vine ripened
  ½ onion, white, large, thinly sliced
  7 fresh basil leaves
  1 t balsamic vinegar
  2 T olive oil, extra-virgin
  1/8 t sea salt

Instructions:

1. Wash the tomatoes and onions well under cool, running water before preparation. Gently wipe vegetables dry with a clean damp towel.

2. Use a clean damp paper towel to gently wipe off the basil, removing any loose dirt.

3. Using a sharp knife remove stem ends from each tomato.

4. 4. Cut tomatoes into 8 wedges.

5. Roll-up the basil leaves one at a time and cut into thin strips crosswise.

6. Combine the vegetables into one bowl and gently toss until well combined.

7. Drizzle with the vinegar and oil and season with salt.

8. Let rest for 20 minutes at room temperature. If made ahead, cover and refrigerate until 20 minutes before service. Tomatoes always taste the best when served at room temperature. Serve at room temperature.

Serving size: ½ cup

Calories	Fiber (g)	Carbs (g)	Protein (g)	Fat (g)
46	1	3	1	4
Chol (mg)	Sodium (mg)	Iron (mg)	Calcium (mg)	Potassium (mg)
0	40	0	1	162

U is for Pineapple Coconut Upside Down Cake

Yield: 9

Enjoy this fabulous cake that is ingredient intense. Read the directions thoroughly making sure you have everything you need before starting. Save the pineapple juice for use in the pot roast recipe.

Oven temperature: 350°F or 177°C

Equipment: oven, measuring cups and spoons, 3-quart mixing bowl, hand mixer, 8-inch round baking pan, oven mitts, large plate, knife

Ingredients:

  1/2 c brown sugar, packed

  2 T butter, unsalted

  15¼ oz can pineapple tidbits, drained

  2 c unbleached all purpose flour

  1 T flax seed meal

  ½ c sugar, granulated

  1½ t baking powder

  ¼ t salt

  ¾ c milk, skim

  1/3 c canola oil

  2 egg whites, jumbo, raw

  1 t vanilla extract

  1 t coconut extract

Instructions:

Preheat oven to 350°F. Cover bottom of baking pan with waxed paper.

1. Combine melted butter and brown sugar mixing until smooth.

2. Pour in bottom of pan.

3. Place the well-drained pineapple in a single layer on top the sugar mixture, set aside.

4. In a mixing bowl combine the remaining ingredients and beat using a hand mixer on low speed for 30 seconds, scraping sides of bowl half-way through.

5. Beat on high speed for 2 minutes, scraping sides of bowl as needed.

6. Gradually pour the cake batter over the pineapple in the baking pan.

7. Bake for about 30 minutes or until a wooden toothpick inserted in the center of the cake comes out clean.

8. Remove cake from oven. Gently flip cake upside down onto an ovenproof plate. Let cake rest inverted with the pan on top for about 7 minutes. Gently remove pan. Serve warm.

Serving size: 1/9th cake

Calories	Fiber (g)	Carbs (g)	Protein (g)	Fat (g)
288	1	44	4	11
Chol (mg)	Sodium (mg)	Iron (mg)	Calcium (mg)	Potassium (mg)
7	171	1	92	133

V is for
Steamed Vegetables—Broccoli

Yield: 2 cups

Use the water from steaming the broccoli in a soup, stew or sauce.

Equipment: 3-quart saucepan with lid, steaming basket, measuring cup

Ingredients:

water

½ lb broccoli, stems and florets cut in 1-2" pieces

Instructions:

1. Fill the bottom of a 3-quart saucepan with 2/3 cup water, lower basket into pan.

2. Heat water to a simmer, add the vegetables to the basket and cover with a lid.

3. Cook on medium heat until just tender, about 6-7 minutes. Broccoli will turn bright green. Remove from heat immediately. Serve hot.

Serving size: ½ cup

Calories	Fiber (g)	Carbs (g)	Protein (g)	Fat (g)
12	1	2	1	0
Chol (mg)	**Sodium (mg)**	**Iron (mg)**	**Calcium (mg)**	**Potassium (mg)**
0	12	0	17	112

W is for Walk the Trail Mix

Yield: 3 cups

Toss together this quick and easy trail mix recipe for a quick energy boost ideal for eating on the go.

Equipment: measuring cup, storage bags

Ingredients:

½ c cherries, dried, not packed

½ c apples, dried, pieces

¼ c apricots, dried

½ c English walnuts, pieces

¼ c sunflower seeds, raw

½ c raisins, not packed

¼ c banana chips

¼ c almonds, whole, raw

Instructions:

Mix all ingredients in a bowl and divide into small storage bags for portion control and portability.

Serving size: ¼ cup

Calories	Fiber (g)	Carbs (g)	Protein (g)	Fat (g)
180	3	24	3	10
Chol (mg)	**Sodium (mg)**	**Iron (mg)**	**Calcium (mg)**	**Potassium (mg)**
0	6	1	32	297

X is for X-tra EZ Energy Bars

Yield: 24 bars

True to its name, this recipe makes a nutritious take-along snack ideal for the lunchbox, gym bag or briefcase. Bars store best in airtight containers.
Source: Adapted from the original recipe by USDA.

Oven temperature: 350°F or 177°C

Equipment: oven, measuring cups, 3-quart saucepan, tablespoon, rimmed cookie sheet, oven mitts, sharp knife, pancake turner

Ingredients:

   non-stick cooking spray

   ½ c brown sugar, packed

   ½ c honey, pasteurized

   1 c peanut butter, chunky style

   3½ c rolled oats, dry

   ½ c raisins, seedless, not packed

   1/3 c dried cranberries, not packed

   ½ c coconut, dried, flaked

Instructions:

Preheat oven to 350°F. Lightly coat baking sheet with non-stick cooking spray, set aside.

1. Over low heat combine honey, brown sugar and peanut butter in a 3-quart saucepan, stirring until melted.

2. Cook until mixture bubbles, stirring often.

3. Immediately remove from heat.

4. Add the remaining ingredients and mix thoroughly.

5. Once cool enough to handle, pour the mixture onto a prepared baking sheet and evenly pat down to ½-inch thick.

6. Bake for 25 minutes. Bars will turn a light golden color when done.

7. Remove from oven. Let cool for about 10 minutes, cut into 24 portions. Serve at room temperature.

Serving size: 1 bar

Calories	Fiber (g)	Carbs (g)	Protein (g)	Fat (g)
163	3	24	4	7
Chol (mg)	Sodium (mg)	Iron (mg)	Calcium (mg)	Potassium (mg)
0	60	1	16	160

Y is for Baked Yams

Yield: 4

This simple recipe produces moist, luscious baked yams. Sometimes mistaken as a sweet potato, yams are less sweet than sweet potatoes and originate from a different botanical family.

Oven temperature: 350°F or 177°C

Equipment: oven, vegetable brush, fork, oven mitts

Ingredients:

2—8 oz yams
non-stick cooking spray

Instructions:

Preheat oven to 350°F.

1. Scrub yams well under cool, running water to remove dirt and debris.

2. Wipe dry with a clean, dry towel. Spray yams with non-stick cooking spray and pierce with a fork.

3. Bake in oven for about 45-50 minutes or until yams give to gentle pressure. Remove from the oven and cut into equal halves. Serve hot.

Serving size: ½ yam

Calories	Fiber (g)	Carbs (g)	Protein (g)	Fat (g)
135	5	31	2	1
Chol (mg)	**Sodium (mg)**	**Iron (mg)**	**Calcium (mg)**	**Potassium (mg)**
0	9	1	16	761

Z is for Reduced Fat Zucchini Bread

Yield: 2 loaves

The delicate flavor of zucchini squash is perfect for using in quick bread recipes.

Source: Adapted from the original recipe by Ginny Roach.

Oven temperature: 350°F or 177°C

Equipment: two 9 inch x 5 inch loaf pans, oven, measuring cups, measuring spoons, 3-quart mixing bowl, shredder, hand mixer, 1 loaf pan, oven mitts, serrated knife, cooling rack, timer

Ingredients:

non-stick cooking spray

2/3 c buttermilk, low-fat (1%)

1 c sugar, granulated

6 egg whites, large, raw (from 6 large eggs)

1/3 c canola oil

1 t vanilla extract

3 c unbleached all purpose flour

1 T cinnamon, ground

½ t nutmeg, ground

1 t baking soda

1 t baking powder

¼ t salt

2 c zucchini, raw, shredded

½ c raisins, seedless, not packed

1/3 c English walnuts, chopped

Instructions:

Preheat oven to 350°F. Spray loaf pans with cooking spray and set aside.

1. In a large mixing bowl combine sugar, eggs, buttermilk, oil and vanilla.

2. In a separate bowl combine flour, cinnamon, nutmeg, baking soda, baking powder, and salt.

3. Add the dry ingredients to the liquid ingredients and mix well.

4. Wash zucchini under cool, running water removing all dirty, debris including stem. Shred zucchini by rubbing it back and forth against a vegetable shredder that has sharp, medium pores.

5. Stir the zucchini, raisins, and walnuts into the batter, gently.

6. Divide batter evenly among the two prepared loaf pans.

7. Bake for 55 to 65 minutes or until a wooden toothpick inserted in the center of a loaf comes out clean.

8. Remove loaves from the oven and leave in pan to cool for 10 minutes.

9. Gently loosen the loaves from the sides of the pan with a knife and remove from the pans. Let the bread cool completely on a wire cooling rack.

10. Cut into ½ inch slices using a serrated knife. Serve warm.

Serving size: 1/12th loaf

Calories	Fiber (g)	Carbs (g)	Protein (g)	Fat (g)
146	1	24	3	4
Chol (mg)	**Sodium (mg)**	**Iron (mg)**	**Calcium (mg)**	**Potassium (mg)**
0	120	1	30	99

Buen Appetito!

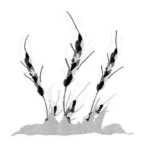

BIBLIOGRAPHY

Chapter 1

1. Prochaska J, DiClemente C. Stages and processes of self-change in smoking: toward an integrative model of change. *J Consult Clin Psych.* 1983;51(3):390-5.

Chapter 2

1. Nitzke S, Freeland-Graves J. Position of the American Dietetic Association: total diet approach to communicating food and nutrition information. *J Am Diet Assoc.* 2007;107:1224-1232.

2. Craig WJ, Mangels AR. Position of the American Dietetic Association: vegetarian diets. *J Am Diet Assoc.* 2009;109:1266-82.

3. Position of The American Dietetic Association: Functional foods. *J Am Diet Assoc.* 2009;109;4:735-746.

4. US Department of Agriculture, Food and Nutrition Service. Building blocks for fun and healthy meals, appendix d: major nutrients. Food and Nutrition Services Web site. http://www.fns. usda.gov/tn/Resources/appendd.pdf. Published 2000. Accessed January 5, 2011.

5. Duyff, RL. Fluids: how much is enough. In: *American Dietetic Association Complete Food and Nutrition Guide.* 3rd ed. Hoboken, NJ: John Wiley and Sons Inc; 2006:156.

6. National Institutes of Health, Office of Dietary Supplements. Dietary supplement fact sheets. Office of Dietary Supplements Web site. http://ods.od.nih.gov/factsheets/list-all/. Published August 24, 2009. Accessed January 5, 2011.

7. US Department of Agriculture, Agricultural Research Service, Nutrient Data Laboratory, National Nutrient Database for Standard Reference, Release 23. US Department of Agriculture, Agricultural Research Service Web site. http://www.ars.usda. gov/ba/bhnrc/ndl. Published October 2010. Accessed January 5, 2011.

8. Panel on Micronutrients, Subcommittees on Upper Reference Levels of Nutrients and of Interpretation and Use of Dietary Reference Intakes, and the Standing Committee on the Scientific Evaluation of Dietary Reference Intakes. Chapter 10: manganese. US Department of Agriculture, National Agriculture Library Web site. http://www.nal.usda.gov/fnic/DRI/DRI_Vitamin_A/ vitamin_a_full_report.pdf. Published 2001. Accessed January 5, 2011.

9. International Food Information Council Foundation (IFIC). Background on functional foods. IFIC's Food Insight: Your Nutrition and Food Safety Web site. http://www.foodinsight.org/

Resources/Detail.aspx?topic=Hoja_de_datos_Dioxinas_dieta_y_
salud. Accessed February 13, 2011.

10. International Food Information Council Foundation (IFIC).
     Functional foods fact sheet: antioxidants. IFIC's Food Insight:
     Your Nutrition and Food Safety Web site. http://www.
     foodinsight.org/Resources/Detail.aspx?topic=Functional_
     Foods_Fact_Sheet_Antioxidants. Published October 15, 2009.
     Accessed January 24, 2011.

11. National Institutes of Health, National Center for
     Complementary and Alternative Medicine (NCCAM). NCCAM
     Web site. http://nccam.nih.gov/health/probiotics/introduction.
     htm. Accessed February 11, 2011.

Chapter 3

1. The Report of the Dietary Guidelines Advisory Committee
    on Dietary Guidelines for Americans, 2010. US Department
    of Agriculture and US Department of Health and Human
    Services Web site. http://www.cnpp.usda.gov/Publications/
    DietaryGuidelines/2010/DGAC/Report/A-ExecSummary.pdf.
    Accessed June 11, 2011.

2. US Department of Agriculture. Grains: what foods are in
    the grains group? ChooseMyPlate.gov Web site. http://www.
    choosemyplate.gov/foodgroups/grains.html. Updated May 31,
    2011. Accessed June 5, 2011.

3. Margen, S and the Editors of the University of California at
    Berkeley WELLNESS LETTER. Nutrition basics: fiber—strong
    links to disease prevention. In: *The Wellness Encyclopedia of Food
    and Nutrition.* New York, NY: Random House, Inc; 1992:19-21.

4.   Kobuszewski, AM. Relax with fiber: fiber defined. *Albertsons Smart Eating Guide.* Boise, ID: Albertsons; 2003. Brochure.

5.   Slavin JL. Position of the American Dietetic Association: health implications of dietary fiber. J Am Diet Assoc. 2008;108:1716-31.

6.   Duyff, RL. "Vegging out" the healthy way. In: *American Dietetic Association Complete Food and Nutrition Guide.* 3rd ed. Hoboken, NJ: John Wiley and Sons Inc; 2006:517-18.

Table 3.1 Daily recommended total dietary fiber intake. Institute of Medicine, Food and Nutrition Board. *Dietary Reference Intakes: Energy, Carbohydrates, Fiber, Fatty Acids, Cholesterol, Protein and Amino Acids.* National Academy of Science Web site. http://www.iom.edu/Reports/2002/Dietary-Reference-Intakes-for-Energy-Carbohydrate-Fiber-Fat-Fatty-Acids-Cholesterol-Protein-and-Amino-Acids.aspx. Published September 5, 2002. Accessed November 29, 2010.

Table 3.2 Estimated dietary fiber content of various foods. US Department of Agriculture, Agricultural Research Service, Nutrient Data Laboratory, National Nutrient Database for Standard Reference, Release 23. US Department of Agriculture, Agricultural Research Service Web site. http://www.ars.usda.gov/main/site_main. htm?modecode=12-35-45-00. Published October 1, 2010. Accessed November 29, 2010.

Chapter 4

1.   *Dietary Guidelines for Americans, 2010.* 7th ed. Washington, DC: US Depts of Agriculture and Health and Human Services; 1312011:33-39.

2.   US Department of Agriculture. Protein foods: why is it important to make lean or low-fat choices from the protein foods group? ChooseMyPlate.gov Web site. http://www. choosemyplate.gov/foodgroups/proteinfoods_why.html. Updated May 31, 2011. Accessed June 5, 2011.

3.   The Report of the Dietary Guidelines Advisory Committee on Dietary Guidelines for Americans, 2010. US Department of Agriculture and US Department of Health and Human Services Web site. http://www.cnpp.usda.gov/Publications/

DietaryGuidelines/2010/DGAC/Report/A-ExecSummary.pdf. Accessed June 11, 2011.

4. US Department of Agriculture. Protein foods: what foods are in the protein foods group? ChooseMyPlate.gov Web site. http://www.choosemyplate.gov/foodgroups/proteinfoods.html. Updated May 31, 2011. Accessed June 5, 2011.

5. US Department of Agriculture. Protein foods: how much food from the protein foods group is needed daily? ChooseMyPlate. gov Web site. http://www.choosemyplate.gov/foodgroups/ proteinfoods_amount.aspx. Updated May 31, 2011. Accessed June 5, 2011.

6. American Cancer Society. Stomach cancer: what are the risk factors for stomach cancer? American Cancer Society Web site. http://www.cancer.org/Cancer/StomachCancer/DetailedGuide/ stomach-cancer-risk-factors. Published October 21, 2010. Accessed January 19, 2011.

Chapter 5

1. *Dietary Guidelines for Americans, 2010.* 7th ed. Washington, DC: US Depts of Agriculture and Health and Human Services; 1312011:20-32.

2. National Institutes of Health, Office of Dietary Supplements. Dietary supplement fact sheets. Office of Dietary Supplements Web site. http://ods.od.nih.gov/pdf/factsheets/ Omega3FattyAcidsandHealth.pdf. Accessed January 20, 2011.

3.   US Food and Drug Administration. Revealing trans fats. Federal Citizen Information Center of the U.S. General Services Administration Web site. http://www.pueblo.gsa.gov/cic_text/food/reveal-fats/reveal-fats.htm. Accessed April 2, 2011.

4.   The Dietary Guidelines for Americans, 2005. The chapter on fats. US Department of Agriculture and US Department of Health and Human Services Web site. http://www.health.gov/dietaryguidelines/dga2005/document/html/chapter6.htm. Published 2005. Accessed January 21, 2011.

5.   National Heart, Lung, and Blood Institute. Your guide to lowering your cholesterol with therapeutic lifestyle change (TLC). Bethesda, MD: US Department of Health and Human Services, National Institutes of Health. 122005. NIH publication 06-5235.

6.   Institute of Medicine. Dietary Reference Intakes for Calcium and Vitamin D. Washington, DC: National Academies Press; 2010.

7.   US Food and Drug Administration. Food: what you need to know about mercury in fish and shellfish. US Food and Drug Administration Web site. http://www.fda.gov/Food/ResourcesForYou/Consumers/ucm110591.htm. Published November 23, 2009. Accessed January 21, 2011.

Table 5.1 Percentage of fat related to calories consumed daily. Kobuszewski, AM. San Leandro, CA: AnitaBeHealthy; 2011.

Table 5.2 Selected seafood and related energy and nutrient contents. US Department of Agriculture, Agricultural Research Service, Nutrient Data Laboratory, National Nutrient Database for Standard Reference, Release 23. US Department of Agriculture, Agricultural Research Service Web site. http://www.ars.usda.gov/ba/bhnrc/ndl. Published October 2010. Accessed October 17, 2010.

Chapter 6

1. US Department of Agriculture. Vegetables: why is it important to eat vegetables? ChooseMyPlate.gov Web site. http://www.choosemyplate.gov/foodgroups/vegetables_why.html. Updated May 31, 2011. Accessed June 5, 2011.

2. US Department of Agriculture. Fruits: why is it important to eat fruit? ChooseMyPlate.gov Web site. http://www.choosemyplate.gov/foodgroups/fruits_why.html. Updated May 31, 2011. Accessed June 5, 2011.

3. *Dietary Guidelines for Americans, 2010.* 7th ed. Washington, DC: US Depts of Agriculture and Health and Human Services; 1312011:35.

4. Adapted from the vegetables: what counts as a cup of vegetables section of US Department of Agriculture: ChooseMyPlate.gov Web site. http://www.choosemyplate.gov/foodgroups/vegetables_counts.html. Updated May 31, 2011. Accessed June 5, 2011.

5. Adapted from the fruits: what counts as a cup of fruit section of US Department of Agriculture: ChooseMyPlate.gov Web site. http://www.choosemyplate.gov/foodgroups/fruits_counts.html. Updated May 31, 2011. Accessed June 5, 2011.

6. US Department of Agriculture. Vegetables: tips to help you eat vegetables. ChooseMyPlate.gov Web site. http://www.choosemyplate.gov/foodgroups/vegetables_tips.html. Updated May 31, 2011. Accessed June 5, 2011.

7.   US Department of Agriculture. Fruits: tips to help you eat fruits. ChooseMyPlate.gov Web site. http://www.choosemyplate.gov/foodgroups/fruits_tips.html. Updated May 31, 2011. Accessed June 5, 2011.

8.   National Institutes of Health, National Libraries of Medicine. Definition and contribution to health of antioxidants. MedlinePlus Web site. http://www.nlm.nih.gov/medlineplus/antioxidants.html. Accessed December 14, 2010.

9.   US Department of Agriculture, Agricultural Research Service. Phytonutrients take center stage. US Department of Agriculture, Agricultural Research Service Web site. http://www.ars.usda.gov/is/ar/archive/dec99/stage1299.htm. Published November 1999. Accessed December 14, 2010.

10.   Baghurst, K. The health benefits of citrus fruits, page 14. *Commonwealth Scientific and Industrial Research Organization, Health Sciences and Nutrition.* Citrus Australia Web site. http://www.citrusaustralia.com.au/PDFs/projects/Health_Benefits_of_Citrus_Final_Report.pdf. Published 2003. Accessed December 14, 2010.

11.   Chen CYO, Blumberg JB. Phytochemical composition of nuts. *Asia Pac J Clin Nutr.* 2008;17(S1):329-332.

12.   Duyff, RL. Phytonutrients: a 'crop' for good health. In: *American Dietetic Association Complete Food and Nutrition Guide.* 3rd ed. Hoboken, NJ: John Wiley and Sons Inc; 2006:109-111.

13.   International Food Information Council Foundation (IFIC). Functional foods fact sheet: antioxidants. IFIC's Food Insight: Your Nutrition and Food Safety Web site. http://www.foodinsight.org/Resources/Detail.aspx?topic=Functional_Foods_Fact_Sheet_Antioxidants. Published October 15, 2009. Accessed January 24, 2011.

14. US Department of Agriculture, Agricultural Research Service. USDA database for the proanthocyanidin content of selected foods, Release 2.1. US Department of Agriculture, Agricultural Research Service Web site. http://www.ars.usda.gov/Services/docs.htm?docid=5843. Published 2007. Accessed May 19, 2011.

15. Garden-Robinson J. What color is your food? Taste a rainbow of fruits and vegetables for better health. North Dakota State University Agriculture and University Extension Web site. http://www.ag.ndsu.edu/pubs/yf/foods/fn595w.htm. Revised February 2009; FN-595. Accessed December 14, 2010.

16. American Dietetic Association. Paint your palate with color. American Dietetic Association Web site. http://www.eatright.org/Public/content.aspx?id=97&terms=phytonutrient. Published July 2008. Accessed December 23, 2010.

17. US Department of Agriculture, Agricultural Research Service. What is vitamin C and what does it do? US Department of Agriculture, Agricultural Research Service Web site. http://ods.od.nih.gov/factsheets/Vitaminc-Consumer/#h3. Updated July 7, 2010. Accessed December 15, 2010.

18. Margen, S and the Editors of the University of California at Berkeley WELLNESS LETTER. Legumes, nuts and seeds. In: *The Wellness Encyclopedia of Food and Nutrition.* New York, NY: Random House, Inc; 1992:358-370.

19. US Department of Agriculture, Agricultural Research Service, Nutrient Data Laboratory, National Nutrient Database for Standard Reference, Release 23. US Department of Agriculture, Agricultural Research Service Web site. http://www.ars.usda.gov/ba/bhnrc/ndl. Published October 2010. Accessed December 15, 2010.

20.   Kobuszewski, AM. The truth about tea and your health. *Albertsons Smart Eating Guide.* Boise, ID: Albertsons; 2004. Brochure.

21.   Kobuszewski, AM. Tea—drink and thrive. *Dietitians in Integrative and Functional Medicine (DIFM).* American Dietetic Association, Chicago, IL. 2005;8:1:9-11.

22.   Wolke RL. *What Einstein Told His Cook: Kitchen Science Explained.* New York, NY: W W Norton & Company, Inc; 2002.

23.   The Oolong Tea. Information on oolong tea. The Oolong Tea Web site. http://www.oolongtea.org/e/index.html. Accessed December 15, 2010.

24.   The Tea Association of the USA. About tea. The Tea Association of the USA Web site. http://www.teausa.com/general/501g.cfm. Accessed December 15, 2010.

25.   Cao G, Sofic E. Prior RL. Antioxidants capacity of tea and common vegetables. The US Department of Agriculture, National Agricultural Library's Digital Repository Web site. http://ddr.nal.usda.gov/bitstream/10113/65/1/IND20576745.pdf . *J Agric Food Chem.* 1996;44:3426-3431.

26.   The Tea Association of the USA. An overview of the health benefits of tea. The Tea Association of the USA Web site. http://www.teausa.com/general/teaandhealth/218g.cfm#ohealth. Accessed December 15, 2010.

27.   Gisslen W. Coffee and tea. In: *Professional Cooking.* New York, NY: John Wiley and Sons, Inc; 1983:513-516.

Chapter 7

1. US Department of Agriculture. The basics: food groups. ChooseMyPlate.gov Web site. http://www.choosemyplate.gov/foodgroups/index.html. Updated June 4, 2011. Accessed June 23, 2011.

2. National Institutes of Health, National Institute on Aging. Eating healthy after 50. National Institute on Aging Web site. http://www.nia.nih.gov/healthinformation/publications/healthyeating.htm. Updated October 5, 2010. Accessed December 17, 2010.

3. *Dietary Guidelines for Americans, 2010.* 7th ed. Washington, DC: US Depts of Agriculture and Health and Human Services; 1312011:4.

4. US Department of Health and Human Services, National Institutes of Health, and National Heart, Lung, and Blood Institute. Diseases and conditions Index: DASH eating plan key points. National Heart, Lung, and Blood Institute Web site. http://www.nhlbi.nih.gov/health/dci/Diseases/dash/dash_summary.html. Accessed January 27, 2011.

5. Kobuszewski, AM. Food after 50: eating for healthy living after 50! *Lucky Stores: The Shopper's Guide to Smart Eating.* San Leandro, CA: American Stores; 1999. Brochure.

6. National Institutes of Health, National Institute on Aging. Exercise and physical activity: getting fit for life. National Institute on Aging Web site. http://www.nia.nih.gov/HealthInformation/Publications/exercise.htm. Updated May 28, 2010. Accessed December 17, 2010.

7. US Department of Health and Human Services, Centers for Disease Control and Prevention. Preventing the flu: good health habits can help stop germs. Centers for Disease Control and Preventions Web site. http://www.cdc.gov/flu/protect/habits. htm. Updated September 27, 2010. Accessed December 17, 2010.

Table 7.1 Calories consumed matched to calories used. National Institutes of Health, National Institute on Aging. Eating healthy after 50. National Institute on Aging Web site. http://www.nia.nih.gov/healthinformation/publications/healthyeating.htm. Updated October 5, 2010. Accessed October 28, 2010.

Chapter 8

1. US Department of Health and Human Services, National Institute of Health, National Heart, Lung, and Blood Institute. We can: families finding the balance. Bethesda, MD: US Department of Health and Human Services, National Institutes of Health. 62005. NIH publication 05-5273. National Heart, Lung, and Blood Institute Web site. http://www.nhlbi.nih.gov/ health/public/heart/obesity/wecan_mats/parent_hb_en.pdf. Accessed December 19, 2010.

2. US Department of Agriculture. Food groups: grains group, vegetable group, fruit group, dairy group, protein foods group. ChooseMyPlate.gov Web site. http://www.choosemyplate.gov/ foodgroups/index.html. Updated May 31, 2011. Accessed June 5, 2011.

3. US Department of Health and Human Services, US Food and Drug Administration. Guidance for industry, a food labeling guide, definitions of nutrient content claims. US Food and Drug Administration Web site. http://www.fda. gov/Food/GuidanceComplianceRegulatoryInformation/ GuidanceDocuments/FoodLabelingNutrition/ FoodLabelingGuide/ucm064911.htm. Updated December 9, 2010. Accessed February 4, 2011.

4. US Food and Drug Administration. Guidance for industry, a food labeling guide, additional requirements for nutrient content claims. US Food and Drug Administration Web site. http://www.fda.gov/Food/GuidanceComplianceRegulatoryInformation/GuidanceDocuments/FoodLabelingNutrition/FoodLabelingGuide/ucm064916.htm. Published April 2008. Accessed February 4, 2011.

5. Baker S, Sutherland B. Mitchell R. Rogers K. Lesson plan two: plan, shop, save. In: *Eating Smart—Being Active.* Fort Collins, CO: Colorado State University Extension; 2007.

6. US Department of Health and Human Services, National Institute of Health, National Institute of Diabetes and Digestive and Kidney Diseases. Weight-control information network: statistics related to overweight and obesity. National Institute of Health, National Heart, Lung, and Blood Institute Web site. http://www.win.niddk.nih.gov/statistics/index.htm. Accessed on December 19, 2010.

7. US Department of Health and Human Services, Centers for Disease Control and Prevention. Defining Overweight and Obesity. Centers for Disease Control and Prevention Web site. http://www.cdc.gov/obesity/defining.html. Accessed April 23, 2011.

8. US Department of Health and Human Services, National Institutes of Health, and National Heart, Lung, and Blood Institute. What does body mass index mean? National Heart, Lung, and Blood Institute Web site. http://www.nhlbi.nih.gov/health/dci/Diseases/obe/obe_diagnosis.html. Accessed December 19, 2010.

9.   US Department of Health and Human Services, National Institutes of Health, and National Heart, Lung, and Blood Institute. What does body mass index mean? National Heart, Lung, and Blood Institute Web site. http://www.nhlbi.nih.gov/health/dci/Diseases/obe/obe_treatments.html. Accessed January 30, 2011.

10. US Department of Health and Human Services, National Institute of Health, National Heart, Lung, and Blood Institute, and Indian Health Service. Honoring the gift of heart health: a heart health educator's manual. National Institute of Health, National Heart, Lung, and Blood Institute Web site. http://www.nhlbi.nih.gov/health/prof/heart/other/aian_manual/ak_manual.pdf. Accessed on February 4, 2011.

11. Sports, Cardiovascular, and Wellness Nutrition—Practice Group of the American Dietetic Association registered dietitians. Nutrition fact sheet: exercise hydration. Sports, Cardiovascular, Wellness Nutrition Web site. http://www.scandpg.org/local/resources/files/2009/SD-USA_Fact_Sheet_Exercise_Hydration_Apr09.pdf. Published April 2009. Accessed February 4, 2011.

12. US Department of Health and Human Services, Centers for Disease Control and Prevention. Commercially bottled water. Centers for Disease Control and Prevention Web site. http://www.cdc.gov/healthywater/drinking/bottled/index.html. Updated April 16, 2010. Accessed December 19, 2010.

13. Environmental Protection Agency, Office of Water. Protect your drinking water for life. Office of Water Web site. http://water.epa.gov/action/protect/. Accessed February 4, 2011.

14. US Department of Agriculture, Agricultural Research Service, Nutrient Data Laboratory, National Nutrient Database for Standard Reference, Release 23. US Department of Agriculture, Agricultural Research Service Web site. http://www.ars.usda.gov/ba/bhnrc/ndl. Published October 2010. Accessed February 4, 2011.

15. US Department of Agriculture, Food Safety and Inspection Services. Food safety information: food safety while hiking, camping and boating. Food Safety and Inspection Services Web site. http://www.fsis.usda.gov/PDF/Food_Safety_While_Hiking_Camping_Boating.pdf. Revised May 2007. Accessed December 19, 2010.

16. Kobuszewski, AM. Stress and nutrition. *Albertsons Smart Eating Guide*. Boise, ID: Albertsons; 2001. Brochure.

17. Liebgold, H. Control your breath, control your life. In: *Liebgold H, More Phobease Revisited: Understanding and Curing Anxiety, Panic, Phobias and Obsessive Complusive Disorders (Book 2)*. Hercules, CA: Liebro Company; 2000:15-16.

18. Rampersaud GC, Pereira MA, Girard BL, Adams J, Metzl JD. Breakfast habits, nutritional status, body weight, and academic performance in children and adolescents. J Am Diet Assoc. 2005;105:743-60.

Table 8.1 Body Mass Index values for adults. US Department of Health and Human Services, National Institutes of Health, and National Heart, Lung, and Blood Institute. National Heart, Lung, and Blood Institute Web site. http://www.nhlbi.nih.gov/health/dci/Diseases/obe/obe_diagnosis.html. Accessed February 28, 2011.

Table 8.2 Estimated calories used during 30 minutes of selected activities. US Department of Health and Human Services, National Institutes of Health, and National Heart, Lung, and Blood Institute. National Heart, Lung, and Blood Institute Web site. http://www.nhlbi.nih.gov/health/prof/heart/other/aian_manual/ak_manual.pdf. Accessed October 30, 2010.

Chapter 9

1. Smith MA. Stepping stones to perennial garden design: site assessment and sunlight. University of Illinois at Urbana-Champaign Extension Web site. http://web.extension.illinois.edu/gardendesign/assessment_sunlight.html. Published 2010. Accessed February 2, 2011.

2. Wester R, Kehr A. Fassuliotis G. Gomez R. Growing vegetables in the home garden. Michigan State University Extension Web site. http://agnic.msu.edu/hgpubs/modus/morefile/hg202_85.pdf. Published 1972. Revised 1985. Accessed February 8, 2011.

3. Pleasant B. Great ways to water. In: *Gardening Essentials.* Minnetonka, MN: National Home Gardening Club; 1999:36–37.

4. US Department of Agriculture, Natural Resource Conservation Service. Home and garden tips: lawn and garden care—alternatives to pesticides and chemicals. Natural Resources Conservation Service Web site. http://www.nrcs.usda.gov/feature/highlights/homegarden/lawn.html. Accessed February 8, 2011.

5. US Department of Health and Human Services, Centers for Disease Control and Prevention. Family health: gardening health and safety tips. Centers for Disease Control and Prevention Web site. http://www.cdc.gov/family/gardening. Updated September 1, 2010. Accessed February 8, 2011.

Table 9.1 Natural pest repellents. US Department of Agriculture, Natural Resource Conservation Service. Home and garden tips: lawn and garden care—alternatives to pesticides and chemicals. Natural Resources Conservation Service Web site. http://www.nrcs.usda.gov/feature/highlights/homegarden/lawn.html. Accessed February 2, 2011.

Chapter 10

1. Gisslen W. Basic cooking principles. In: *Professional Cooking.* New York, NY: John Wiley and Sons, Inc; 1983:51-61.

2. Baker S, Sutherland B, Mitchell R, Rogers K. *Eating Smart— Being Active.* Fort Collins, CO: Colorado State University Extension; 2007.

3. US Department of Agriculture. Protein foods: tips to help you make wise choices from the protein foods group. ChooseMyPlate.gov Web site. http://www.choosemyplate.gov/foodgroups/proteinfoods_tips.html. Updated May 31, 2011. Accessed June 5, 2011.

4. US Department of Agriculture. Fruits: why is it important to eat fruit? ChooseMyPlate.gov Web site. http://www.choosemyplate.gov/foodgroups/fruits_why.html. Updated May 31, 2011. Accessed June 4, 2011.

5. US Department of Agriculture. Vegetables: why is it important to eat vegetables? ChooseMyPlate.gov Web site. http://www.choosemyplate.gov/foodgroups/vegetables_why.html. Updated May 31, 2011. Accessed June 5, 2011.

6. United States Department of Agriculture, Food Safety and Inspection Service (FSIS). Kitchen companion: your safe food handbook. FSIS Web site. http://www.fsis.usda.gov/PDF/Kitchen_Companion.pdf. Accessed February 9, 2011.

Table 10.1 In-season vegetables and fruits. Baker S, Sutherland B, Mitchell R, Rogers K. *Eating Smart—Being Active.* Fort Collins, CO: Colorado State University Extension; 2007.

Table 10.2 Safe minimum internal food temperatures. United States Department of Agriculture, Food Safety and Inspection Service (FSIS). Kitchen companion: your safe food handbook. FSIS Web site. http://www.fsis.usda.gov/PDF/Kitchen_Companion.pdf. Accessed February 9, 2011.

Appendices

Appendix A
US Department of Agriculture, Food and Nutrition Service. Read it before you eat it poster in the team nutrition resource library. Food and Nutrition Service Team Nutrition Web site. http://teamnutrition.usda.gov/Resources/read_it.html. Printed 2006. Revised April 2007. Accessed June 4, 2011.

Appendix B
US Department of Agriculture. Dietary guidelines 2010 selected messages for consumers. ChooseMyPlate.gov Web site. http://www.choosemyplate.gov/downloads/MyPlate/SelectedMessages.pdf. Published June 2011. Accessed June 4, 2011.

Appendix C
US Department of Health and Human Services, National Institutes of Health, and National Heart, Lung, and Blood Institute. What does body mass index mean? National Heart, Lung, and Blood Institute Web site. http://www.nhlbi.nih.gov/health/dci/Diseases/obe/obe_diagnosis.html. Accessed June 4, 2011.

Appendix D
The Dietary Guidelines for Americans, 2005. Toolkit for health professionals. US Department of Agriculture and US Department of Health and Human Services Web site. http://www.health.gov/dietaryguidelines/dga2005/toolkit/Worksheets/ShoppingList.pdf. Accessed June 4, 2011.

Appendix E
Adapted from cooking terms section of Kansas State University Research & Extension Family Nutrition Program: Kidz a cookin' where cooking is fun Web site. http://www.kidsacookin.ksu.edu/Site.aspx?page=Terms. Accessed February 22, 2011.

Appendix F
Dairy Council of California. Meal planning made simple: substitutions. Dairy Council of California Meals Matter Web site. http://www.mealsmatter.org/MealPlanning/Substitutions/. Accessed June 4, 2011.

Appendix G

Dairy Council of California. Meal planning made simple: conversions. Dairy Council of California Meals Matter Web site. http://www.mealsmatter.org/MealPlanning/ Equivalents/. Accessed June 4, 2011.

Appendix H

1. Brown, A. Flours and flour mixtures. In: *Understanding Food.* 2nd ed. Belmont, CA: Wadsworth/Thomson Learning, Inc; 2004: 408-409.

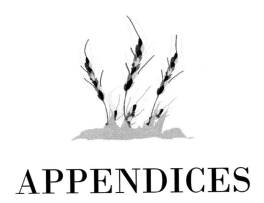

APPENDICES

Appendix A: Label Reading Guide

READ IT *before you EAT IT!*

How many servings are you eating?

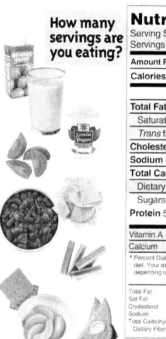

Nutrition Facts
Serving Size 1 cup (228g)
Servings Per Container 2

Amount Per Serving

Calories 250   Calories from Fat 110

	% Daily Value*
Total Fat 12g	18%
Saturated Fat 3g	15%
Trans fat 0g	
Cholesterol 30mg	10%
Sodium 470mg	20%
Total Carbohydrate 31g	10%
Dietary Fiber 0g	0%
Sugars 5g	
Protein 5g	

Vitamin A	4%	•	Vitamin C	2%
Calcium	20%	•	Iron	4%

* Percent Daily Values are based on a 2,000 calorie diet. Your daily values may be higher or lower depending on your calorie needs:

		Calories:	2,000	2,500
Total Fat	Less than		65g	80g
Sat Fat	Less than		20g	25g
Cholesterol	Less than		300mg	300mg
Sodium	Less than		2,400mg	2,400mg
Total Carbohydrate			300g	375g
Dietary Fiber			25g	30g

What food would have this Nutrition Facts label?

Get What You Need!

 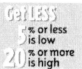

Get LESS
5% or less is low
20% or more is high

Get ENOUGH
5% or less is low
20% or more is high

 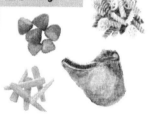

What's the Best Choice for You?
Use the Nutrition Facts Label to Make Choices

Appendix B: Dietary Guidelines for Americans, 2010

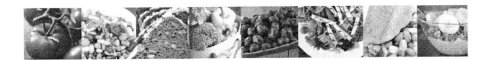

Dietary Guidelines 2010
Selected Messages for Consumers

Take action on the Dietary Guidelines by making changes in these three areas.

Choose steps that work for you and start today.

Balancing Calories

- Enjoy your food, but eat less.
- Avoid oversized portions.

Foods to Increase

- Make half your plate fruits and vegetables.
- Make at least half your grains whole grains.
- Switch to fat-free or low-fat (1%) milk.

Foods to Reduce

- Compare sodium in foods like soup, bread, and frozen meals—and choose the foods with lower numbers.
- Drink water instead of sugary drinks.

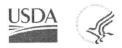

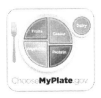

ChooseMyPlate.gov

June 2011

Appendix C: Body Mass Index Table

Body Mass Index Table

Body Weight (pounds)

Height (inches)	Normal						Overweight					Obese						Extreme Obesity																				
BMI	19	20	21	22	23	24	25	26	27	28	29	30	31	32	33	34	35	36	37	38	39	40	41	42	43	44	45	46	47	48	49	50	51	52	53	54
58	91	96	100	105	110	115	119	124	129	134	138	143	148	153	158	162	167	172	177	181	186	191	196	201	205	210	215	220	224	229	234	239	244	248	253	258
59	94	99	104	109	114	119	124	128	133	138	143	148	153	158	163	168	173	178	183	188	193	198	203	208	212	217	222	227	232	237	242	247	252	257	262	267
60	97	102	107	112	118	123	128	133	138	143	148	153	158	163	168	174	179	184	189	194	199	204	209	215	220	225	230	235	240	245	250	255	261	266	271	276
61	100	106	111	116	122	127	132	137	143	148	153	158	164	169	174	180	185	190	195	201	206	211	217	222	227	232	238	243	248	254	259	264	269	275	280	285
62	104	109	115	120	126	131	136	142	147	153	158	164	169	175	180	186	191	196	202	207	213	218	224	229	235	240	246	251	256	262	267	273	278	284	289	295
63	107	113	118	124	130	135	141	146	152	158	163	169	175	180	186	191	197	203	208	214	220	225	231	237	242	248	254	259	265	270	278	282	287	293	299	304
64	110	116	122	128	134	140	145	151	157	163	169	174	180	186	191	197	204	209	215	221	227	232	238	244	250	256	262	267	273	279	285	291	296	302	308	314
65	114	120	126	132	138	144	150	156	162	168	174	180	186	192	198	204	210	216	222	228	234	240	246	252	258	264	270	276	282	288	294	300	306	312	318	324
66	118	124	130	136	142	148	155	161	167	173	179	186	192	198	204	210	216	223	229	235	241	247	253	260	266	272	278	284	291	297	303	309	315	322	328	334
67	121	127	134	140	146	153	159	166	172	178	185	191	198	204	211	217	223	230	236	242	249	255	261	268	274	280	287	293	299	306	312	319	325	331	338	344
68	125	131	138	144	151	158	164	171	177	184	190	197	203	210	216	223	230	236	243	249	256	262	269	276	282	289	295	302	308	315	322	328	335	341	348	354
69	128	135	142	149	155	162	169	176	182	189	196	203	209	216	223	230	236	243	250	257	263	270	277	284	291	297	304	311	318	324	331	338	345	351	358	365
70	132	139	146	153	160	167	174	181	188	195	202	209	216	222	229	236	243	250	257	264	271	278	285	292	299	306	313	320	327	334	341	348	355	362	369	376
71	136	143	150	157	165	172	179	186	193	200	208	215	222	229	236	243	250	257	265	272	279	286	293	301	308	315	322	329	338	343	351	358	365	372	379	386
72	140	147	154	162	169	177	184	191	199	206	213	221	228	235	242	250	258	265	272	279	287	294	302	309	316	324	331	338	346	353	361	368	375	383	390	397
73	144	151	159	166	174	182	189	197	204	212	219	227	235	242	250	257	265	272	280	288	295	302	310	318	325	333	340	348	355	363	371	378	386	393	401	408
74	148	155	163	171	179	186	194	202	210	218	225	233	241	249	256	264	272	280	287	295	303	311	319	326	334	342	350	358	365	373	381	389	396	404	412	420
75	152	160	168	176	184	192	200	208	216	224	232	240	248	256	264	272	279	287	295	303	311	319	327	335	343	351	359	367	375	383	391	399	407	415	423	431
76	156	164	172	180	189	197	205	213	221	230	238	246	254	263	271	279	287	295	304	312	320	328	336	344	353	361	369	377	385	394	402	410	418	426	435	443

Source: Adapted from Clinical Guidelines on the Identification, Evaluation, and Treatment of Overweight and Obesity in Adults: The Evidence Report.

Appendix D: My Shopping List

My Shopping List

Make a shopping list. Include the items you need for your menus and any low-calorie basics you need to restock in your kitchen.

Dairy Case

- [ ] Fat-free (skim) or low-fat (1%) milk
- [ ] Low-fat or reduced fat cottage cheese
- [ ] Fat-free cottage cheese
- [ ] Low-fat or reduced fat cheeses
- [ ] Fat-free or low-fat yogurt
- [ ] Light or diet margarine (tub, squeeze, or spray)
- [ ] Fat-free or reduced fat sour cream
- [ ] Fat-free cream cheese
- [ ] Eggs/egg substitute
- [ ] _____

Breads, Muffins, and Rolls

- [ ] Bread, bagels, or pita bread
- [ ] English muffins
- [ ] Yeast breads (whole wheat, rye, pumpernickel, multi-grain, or raisin)
- [ ] Corn tortillas (not fried)
- [ ] Low-fat flour tortillas
- [ ] Fat-free biscuit mix
- [ ] Rice crackers
- [ ] Challah
- [ ] _____

Cereals, Crackers, Rice, Noodles, and Pasta

- [ ] Plain cereal, dry or cooked
- [ ] Saltines, soda crackers (low-sodium or unsalted tops)
- [ ] Graham crackers
- [ ] Other low-fat crackers
- [ ] Rice (brown, white, etc.)
- [ ] Pasta (noodles, spaghetti)
- [ ] Bulgur, couscous, or kasha
- [ ] Potato mixes (made without fat)
- [ ] Wheat mixes
- [ ] Tabouli grain salad

- [ ] Hominy
- [ ] Polenta
- [ ] Polvillo
- [ ] Hominy grits
- [ ] Quinoa
- [ ] Millet
- [ ] Aramanth
- [ ] Oatmeal
- [ ] _____

Meat Case

- [ ] White meat chicken and turkey (skin off)
- [ ] Fish (not battered)
- [ ] Beef, round or sirloin
- [ ] Extra lean ground beef such as ground round
- [ ] Pork tenderloin
- [ ] 95% fat-free lunch meats or low-fat deli meats
- [ ] _____

Meat Equivalents:

- [ ] Tofu (or bean curd)
- [ ] Beans (see bean list)
- [ ] Eggs/egg substitutes (see dairy list)
- [ ] _____

Fruit (fresh, canned, and frozen)

Fresh Fruit:

- [ ] Apples
- [ ] Bananas
- [ ] Peaches
- [ ] Oranges
- [ ] Pears
- [ ] Grapes
- [ ] Grapefruit
- [ ] Apricots
- [ ] Dried Fruits
- [ ] Cherries
- [ ] Plums

- [ ] Melons
- [ ] Lemons
- [ ] Limes
- [ ] Plantains
- [ ] Mangoes
- [ ] _____

Exotic Fresh Fruit:

- [ ] Kiwi
- [ ] Olives
- [ ] Figs
- [ ] Quinces
- [ ] Currants
- [ ] Persimmons
- [ ] Pomegranates
- [ ] Papaya
- [ ] Zapote
- [ ] Guava
- [ ] Starfruit
- [ ] Litchi nuts
- [ ] Winter melons
- [ ] _____

Canned Fruit (in juice or water):

- [ ] Canned pineapple
- [ ] Applesauce
- [ ] Other canned fruits (mixed or plain)
- [ ] _____

Frozen Fruits (without added sugar):

- [ ] Blueberries
- [ ] Raspberries
- [ ] 100% fruit juice
- [ ] _____

Dried Fruit:

- [ ] Raisins/dried fruit (these tend to be higher in calories than fresh fruit)
- [ ] _____

Vegetables (fresh, canned, and frozen)

Fresh Vegetables:
- ☐ Broccoli
- ☐ Peas
- ☐ Corn
- ☐ Cauliflower
- ☐ Squash
- ☐ Green beans
- ☐ Green leafy vegetables
- ☐ Spinach
- ☐ Lettuce
- ☐ Cabbage
- ☐ Artichokes
- ☐ Cucumber
- ☐ Asparagus
- ☐ Mushrooms
- ☐ Carrots or celery
- ☐ Onions
- ☐ Potatoes
- ☐ Tomatoes
- ☐ Green peppers
- ☐ Chilies
- ☐ _____

Canned Vegetables (low-sodium or no-salt-added):
- ☐ Canned tomatoes
- ☐ Tomato sauce or pasta
- ☐ Other canned vegetables
- ☐ Canned vegetable soup, reduced sodium

Frozen Vegetables: (without added fats):
- ☐ Broccoli
- ☐ Spinach
- ☐ Mixed medley, etc
- ☐ _____

Exotic Fresh Vegetables
- ☐ Okra
- ☐ Eggplant
- ☐ Grape leaves
- ☐ Mustard greens
- ☐ Kale
- ☐ Leeks
- ☐ Bamboo shoots
- ☐ Chinese celery
- ☐ Bok choy
- ☐ Napa cabbage
- ☐ Seaweed

- ☐ Rhubarb
- ☐ _____

Beans and Legumes (if canned, no-salt-added)

- ☐ Lentils
- ☐ Black beans
- ☐ Red beans (kidney beans)
- ☐ Navy beans
- ☐ Black beans
- ☐ Pinto beans
- ☐ Black-eyed peas
- ☐ Fava beans
- ☐ Italian white beans
- ☐ Great white northern beans
- ☐ Chickpeas (garbanzo beans)
- ☐ Dried beans, peas, and lentils (without flavoring packets)
- ☐ _____

Baking Items

- ☐ Flour
- ☐ Sugar
- ☐ Imitation butter (flakes or buds)
- ☐ Non-stick cooking spray
- ☐ Canned evaporated milk– fat-free (skim) or reduced fat (2%)
- ☐ Non-fat dry milk powder
- ☐ Cocoa powder, unsweetened
- ☐ Baking powder
- ☐ Baking soda
- ☐ Cornstarch
- ☐ Unflavored gelatin
- ☐ Gelatin, any flavor (reduced calorie)
- ☐ Pudding mixes (reduced calorie)
- ☐ Angel food cake mix
- ☐ _____

Frozen Foods

- ☐ Fish fillets–unbreaded
- ☐ Egg substitute
- ☐ 100 percent fruit juices (no-sugar-added)
- ☐ Fruits (no-sugar-added)
- ☐ Vegetables (plain)
- ☐ _____

Condiments, Sauces, Seasonings, and Spreads

- ☐ Fat-free or low-fat salad dressings
- ☐ Mustard (Dijon, etc.)
- ☐ Catsup
- ☐ Barbecue sauce
- ☐ Jam, jelly, or honey
- ☐ Spices
- ☐ Flavored vinegars
- ☐ Hoisin sauce and plum sauce
- ☐ Salsa or picante sauce
- ☐ Canned green chilies
- ☐ Soy sauce (low-sodium)
- ☐ Bouillon cubes/granules (low-sodium)
- ☐ _____

Beverages

- ☐ No-calorie drink mixes
- ☐ Reduced calorie juices
- ☐ Unsweetened iced tea
- ☐ Carbonated water
- ☐ Water
- ☐ _____

Nuts and Seeds

- ☐ Almonds, unsalted
- ☐ Mixed nuts, unsalted
- ☐ Peanuts, unsalted
- ☐ Walnuts
- ☐ Sesame seeds
- ☐ Pumpkin seeds, unsalted
- ☐ Sunflower seeds, unsalted
- ☐ Cashews, unsalted
- ☐ Pecans, unsalted
- ☐ _____

Fats and Oils

- ☐ Soft (tub) margarine
- ☐ Mayonnaise, low-fat
- ☐ Canola oil
- ☐ Corn oil
- ☐ Olive oil
- ☐ Safflower oil
- ☐ _____

Appendix E: Cooking Terms

BAKE: To cook by dry heat in an oven. When applied to meats and poultry, this cooking method is called roasting.

BASTE: To brush or spoon a glaze, a sauce, or drippings over a food as it cooks, to add flavor and to help keep the surface moist.

BATTER: A thin mixture of flour and water that can be poured into pan or onto griddle.

BEAT: To vigorously mix one or more ingredients using a brisk up-and-over motion to add air to a mixture. Or, use an electric mixer.

BLANCH: To cover with boiling water for a specific, brief time. A quick cold water rinse often follows the heat. Blanching prevents spoilage during freezing, or loosens skin for peeling.

BLEND: To combine two or more ingredients mixing thoroughly until smooth.

BOIL: To cook in liquid that is heated until bubbles rise to the surface and break. Bubbles form throughout the mixture.

BRAISE: To brown meat in a small amount of fat, then cook slowly in a covered container with a small amount of liquid.

BROIL: To cook by direct heat with the heat source directly over the food. Similar to grilling, however broiling is often done in the kitchen in the oven.

BROWN: To give a cooked surface of a food (such as meat or flour)a brown or toasty appearance by applying high heat. Also occurs during baking and roasting.

CHOP: To cut into small pieces with a sharp knife.

CORE: To remove the seeded, inner portion of a fruit.

CREAM: To rub or work soft fat, often with sugar, against the sides of a bowl or with a whisk or mixer until creamy or fluffy. When making baked goods tiny air pockets form in the fat so the mixture is light and airy.

CUBE: To cut into evenly shaped pieces which are equal on all sides.

CUT: To work fat into dry ingredients with a pastry blender or two knives, with the least possible amount of mixing. Or to use a knife.

DICE: To cut into tiny cubes.

DOUGH: Thick mixture of flour and liquid that can be rolled, kneaded or dropped from a spoon.

DRIZZLE: To pour a light amount, usually from a spoon, over food.

FOLD: To gently incorporate a lighter ingredient into a heavier one by passing a flexible spatula down through a mixture in a bowl, across the bottom, and up over the top until the ingredients are combined. This technique traps air into bubbles in the food, allowing baked goods to rise.

FRY: To cook, usually submerged, in heated fat.

GRATE: To rub foods against grater (a surface with fine to small holes or slits) to divide into small pieces.

KNEAD: To mix using pressing, folding, and stretching motions. Used most commonly in bread baking to develop the gluten in flour.

MARINATE: To immerse a food in an acid mixture to add flavor or tenderize. Some marinades may also incorporate oil in the mixture.

MINCE: To cut or chop into very small pieces.

MIX: To combine two or more ingredients.

PAN-BROIL: To cook uncovered on a hot surface, with little if any added fat. This is usually accomplished using a frying pan or skiller. Fat is poured off as it accumulates.

PAN-FRY: To cook in a small amount of hot fat.

PARBOIL: To boil until partially cooked.

PARE: To cut off the outer covering or skin of vegetables or fruits with a knife or vegetable peeler.

POACH: To cook in a hot liquid.

RECONSTITUTE: To restore a former condition by adding water.

ROAST: To bake.

ROUX: A mixture of melted fat and flour used to make gravy or white sauce.

SAUTÉ: To cook quickly at high heat in a small amount of fat.

SCALD: To bring to a temperature just below boiling so that tiny bubbles form at the edge of the pan.

SCALLOP: To combine pieces of food with a sauce or other liquid and generally finish cooking by baking in the oven.

SEAR: To brown surface of meat quickly with intense heat.

SHRED: To tear food by rubbing across a surface with medium to large holes or slits to make small pieces. May also be accomplished using two forks to separate meat fibers.

SIFT: To mix flour or ingredients with air.

SIMMER: To cook in liquid below the boiling point. Bubbles break before reaching the surface.

STEAM: To cook in steam, with or without pressure.

STIR: To mix with a circular motion.

STIR-FRY: To cook quickly in a small amount of hot fat, stirring constantly.

TOSS: To mix ingredients lightly by lifting and dropping with a spoon, or a spoon and a fork.

WHIP: To beat rapidly to incorporate air.

WHISK: To beat ingredients together, using a wire whip or whisk, until they are well blended.

Source: Adapted cooking terms section of Kansas State University Research & Extension Family Nutrition Program: Kidz a cookin' where cooking is fun Web site. http://www.kidsacookin.ksu.edu/Site.aspx?page=Terms. Accessed February 22, 2011.

Appendix F: Ingredient Substitutions

Substitutions

Stuck without a needed ingredient? Here's a list of common substitutions. Your results may be a little different than usual, especially in baking.

YOGURT is a miracle-worker. Use it instead of...

Mayonnaise	1 tsp Dijon mustard + 1 cup plain yogurt, salt and pepper
Sour cream	Plain or vanilla yogurt + 1 tsp baking soda added to dry ingredients
Cream cheese	Put plain yogurt in a coffee-filter-lined strainer, over a large bowl. Cover and refrigerate 24 hours. Save the whey for baking!
Soup base	2 Tb flour + 1 cup plain yogurt

General Substitutions

1 tsp. Baking powder	1/3 tsp. baking soda + 1/2 tsp. Cream of tartar
1 cup Cake flour	1 cup less 2 Tb. all-purpose flour
1 Tb. Flour for thickening	1 1/2 tsp. cornstarch or arrowroot
1 1/2 tsp. Arrowroot	1 Tb. Flour + 1 1/2 tsp. cornstarch
1 cup self-raising flour	1 cup all-purpose flour plus 1 1/2 tsp. baking powder and 1/2 tsp. salt
Whole eggs	two egg whites for each whole egg + 1 Tb. vegetable oil
1 cup Sour cream	1/3 cup melted butter + 3/4 cup buttermilk
1 cup Buttermilk	1 cup milk mixed with 1 Tb. white vinegar; let stand 10 minutes. Or 1 cup yogurt.
1 oz. Baking chocolate	3 Tb. cocoa + 1 Tb. Shortening or butter
1 cup Dry bread crumbs	3/4 cup fine cracker crumbs
1 tsp. Lemon juice	1/2 tsp. White vinegar
1 clove garlic	1/8 tsp. Garlic powder
1 Tb. Fresh herbs	1 tsp. Dried herbs
1 tsp. Allspice	1/2 tsp cinnamon and 1/2 tsp ground cloves
1 cup honey	1 1/4 cup sugar + 1/4 cup water
1 cup light corn syrup	1 1/4 cup light brown sugar and 1/3 cup water
1 cup dark corn syrup	3/4 cup Light Corn Syrup plus 1/4 cup Molasses OR 1 cup Light Corn Syrup plus 1 Tb. brown sugar

© 2010 Dairy Council of California

Appendix G: Measurement Conversions / Equivalents

Conversions

Measures

3 teaspoons	= 1 Tablespoon
4 Tablespoons	= 1/4 cup
5 Tablespoons and 1 teaspoon	= 1/3 cup
8 Tablespoons	= 1/2 cup
10 Tablespoons and 2 teaspoons	= 2/3 cup
12 Tablespoons	= 3/4 cup
16 Tablespoons	= 1 cup
2 Tablespoons	= 1 liquid ounce
1 cup	= 1/2 pint
2 cups	= 1pint
4 cups	= 1 quart
4 quarts	= 1 gallon

Equivalents

1 lb. Sifted all-purpose flour	= 4 cups
1 lb. White sugar	= 2 1/4-2 1/2 cups
1 lb. Brown sugar, firmly packed	= 2 1/8- 2 1/4 cups
1 lb. Powdered sugar, sifted	= 4 1/2 - 5 cups
1 medium lemon rind, grated	= 1 Tablespoon
1 medium lemon, juiced	= 3 Tablespoons
1 medium orange, juiced	= 1/4 cup juice
4 oz firm cheese (Cheddar, Jack, Swiss)	= 1 cup shredded, lightly packed
3 oz hard cheese (Parmesan, Romano)	= 1/2 cup grated
4 oz almonds or walnut meats	= 1 cup chopped
28 squares saltine (soda) crackers	= 1/4 cup crumbs
16 squares graham crackers	= 1 cup crumbs
24 two-inch vanilla wafers	= 1 cup crumbs
18 two-inch chocolate wafers	= 1 cup crumbs
1 package dry yeast	= 1 Tbsp

Appendix H: The Bread Baking Ceremony

I love to make bread. Now you can enjoy preparing my favorite yeast bread (A+ Honor Rolls) and quick bread (Best Banana Bread) recipes in Chapter 11. The most basic combination of flour, water, salt, and yeast come together after mixing, kneading, fermentation, proofing, shaping, proofing again, and baking is transformed into a loaf of bread. Bread making is the way I acknowledge my physical, emotional, artistic, and spiritual abilities by taking grains planted, sown, grown, harvested, milled, packaged, and eventually delivered to me to use in whatever bread I choose to make. Bread making is a scientific experiment that when done with consistency can result in the most gratifying of human experiences. Edible science.

*   *   *

YEAST TRIVIA: *Yeast (sarcharomyces cerevisiae) has the natural ability to make a gas, carbon dioxide. This is called fermentation. This happens when yeast comes in contact with sugar in the presence of a warm liquid forming carbon dioxide and a tiny bit of alcohol. In the case of bread, the warm temperature provided in the proofing process of bread making helps the yeast grow which in turn causes carbon dioxide to form. This leavening action of carbon dioxide causes the bread dough to rise. The alcohol eventually evaporates during and after the bread is baked. The sugar can be from that naturally found in the flour and/or sugar added to the recipe.*

*   *   *

The different types of yeast include rapid rise, instant and cake yeast. The fermentation temperature for instant dry yeast is between 70-90°F. Above 100°F the reactions slow down. Yeast also provides a very characteristic flavor in bread products.[1]

Once the dough is ready for the dough rising process, also known as proofing, be sure to select the right pan for baking. Why? As yeast bread rises during the proofing and baking processes it expands. If the pan is too small the dough will overflow and if the pan is too large it will flatten out, not rising to its full capacity. The same is true for a quick bread during the baking process. Tall, narrow loaf pans produce taller loaves than short wide pans.

Simply put, yeast bread will rise or proof twice—once as a glob of dough and a second time as a roll or loaf or whatever you've shaped the dough into. A quick bread will rise during the actual baking process. Regardless of which bread you make, preheating the oven is important and will help the dough or batter bake correctly.

Be sure to center your baking pan in the middle of the oven for even cooking. This may require the rearrangement of the metal racks in the oven. Set your timer five minutes shy of the recipe baking time and do an early check on the doneness of the product. When the baking process is complete pull the bread out of the oven and let it cool in the pan as directed, usually on a cooling rack.

Homemade bread typically has a shorter shelf-life than store bought bread that contains preservatives so be sure to place it in an air tight container, or an appropriate bag, after it's thoroughly cooled. Bagging items before they are cool throughout will cause the bread to sweat or draw the water from the inside to the outside as it cools in the confined space of the bag. This will make your bread soggy on the outside and spoil more quickly.

Home baked bread has always been a hit at social gatherings. While it can be time consuming—bread making is always worth the effort. The bench time or the time spent waiting for the dough to rise, is what you'll need to plan for. Enjoy this time-honored ritual often and you will agree it is time well spent.

[1]Source: Brown, Amy. In: *Understanding Food.* 2nd ed. Belmont, CA: Wadsworth/Thomson Learning, Inc; 2004: 408-409.

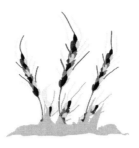

RESOURCE SECTION

The following is a list of websites and other resources that you may use to find additional reliable nutrition and health information.

Accessing General Nutrition Information

American Dietetic Association
www.eatright.org
800-877-1600 or 312-899-0040
120 South Riverside Plaza, Suite 2000
Chicago, IL 60606-6995

Center for Nutrition Policy and Promotion
www.cnpp.usda.gov/
703-305-7600
U.S. Department of Agriculture
3101 Park Center Drive, Suite 1034
Alexandria, VA 22302-1594

Center for Science in the Public Interest
www.cspinet.org
202-332-9110
1875 Connecticut Avenue NW, Suite 300
Washington, D.C. 20009

Dietary Guidelines for Americans, 2010
www.healthierus.gov/dietaryguidelines
240-453-8280
U.S. Department of Health and Human Services
Office of Disease Prevention and Health Promotion
Office of Public Health and Science
Office of the Secretary
1101 Wootton Parkway, Suite LL100
Rockville, MD 20852

Food and Nutrition Information Center

fnic.nal.usda.gov/
301-504-5719
National Agricultural Library
U.S. Department of Agriculture, Room 304
10301 Baltimore Avenue
Beltsville, MD 20705-2351

International Food Information Council (IFIC)

www.foodinsight.org/
202-296-6540
1100 Connecticut Avenue, NW, Suite 430
Washington, D.C. 20036

Institute of Medicine/Food and Nutrition Board

www.iom.edu
202-334-2352
Keck Center W706
500 Fifth Street NW
Washington, D.C. 20001

National Institute of Food and Agriculture

www.csrees.usda.gov/Extension
202-720-4423
U.S. Department of Agriculture
1400 Independence Avenue SW, Stop 2201
Washington, DC 20250-2201

Nutrition, Health, and Food Management Division

www.aafcs.org
800-424-8080 or 703-706-4600
American Association of Family and Consumer Sciences
400 North Columbus Street, Suite 202
Alexandria, VA 22314

Society for Nutrition Education

www.sne.org/

800-235-6690 or 317-328-4627

9100 Purdue Road, Suite 200

Indianapolis, IN 46268

U.S. Government Nutrition Sites

www.nutrition.gov or www.healthfinder.gov (See Quick Guide to Healthy Living, Nutrition, & Fitness)

National Agricultural Library

Food and Nutrition Information Center

10301 Baltimore Avenue

Beltsville, MD 20705-2351

Dietary Supplements

Food and Drug Administration

www.cfsan.fda.gov/~dms/supplmnt.html

888-INFO-FDA (888-463-6332)

10903 New Hampshire Ave

Silver Spring, MD 20993-0002

National Center for Complementary and Alternative Medicine Clearinghouse

nccam.nih.gov/health/supplements/

888-644-6226

P.O. Box 7923

Gaithersburg, MD 20898

U.S. Pharmacopoeia

www.usp.org/USPVerified/dietarySupplements/

800-227-8772

12601 Twinbrook Parkway

Rockville, MD 20852-1790

Educational Materials

Audiovisual/Education Resource Catalogs

Foodplay Productions

www.foodplay.com

800-FOODPLAY (-366-3752)

1 Sunset Ave

Hatfield, MA 01038

Health Edco

www.healthedco.com

800-299-3366

P.O. Box 21207

Waco, TX 76702-1207

NASCO Nutrition Teaching Aids Catalog

www.enasco.com/

800-558-9595

4825 Stoddard Road

Modesto, CA 95356

National Health Video

www.nhv.com

800-543-6803

11312 Santa Monica Boulevard #5

Los Angeles, CA 90025

NCES (Nutrition, Counseling, and Education Services)

www.ncescatalog.com

877-623-7266

1904 East 123rd

Olathe, KS 66061

NEAT Solutions for Healthy Children

www.neatsolutions.com

888-577-NEAT (-6328)

6645 Alhambra Avenue

Martinez, CA 94553

Yummy Designs

www.yummydesigns.com

888-749-8669

P.O. Box 1851

Walla Walla, WA 99362

Food Models

NASCO Nutrition Teaching Aids Catalog

www.nascofa.com

800-558-9595

901 Janesville Avenue

P.O. Box 901

Fort Atkinson, WI 53538-0901

National Dairy Council

www.nationaldairycouncil.org

10255 West Higgins Road, Suite 900

Rosemont, IL 60018

NCES (Nutrition, Counseling and Educational Services)

www.ncescatalog.com

877-623-7266

1904 East 123rd

Olathe, KS 66061

General Resources

Food And Health Communications

www.foodandhealth.com

P.O. Box 266498

Weston, FL 33326

954-385-5328

Health Teacher

www.healthteacher.com

800-514-1362

5200 Maryland Way, Suite 100

Brentwood, TN 37027

Healthy Kids Challenge

www.healthykidschallenge.com

888-259-6287

2 W Road 210

Dighton, KS 67839

Healthy Start

www.Healthy-Start.com

631-549-0010 extension 114

MyPlate (previously MyPyramid)

www.ChooseMyPlate.gov

888-779-7264

USDA Center for Nutrition Policy and Promotion

3101 Park Center Drive, Room 1034

Alexandria, VA 22302-1594

Teach Free

www.teachfree.org

Washington State Dairy Council

www.eatsmart.org

425-744-1616

4201 198th Street, SW,

Lynnwood, WA 98036-6751

Food Allergy/Food Sensitivity

American Academy of Allergy, Asthma, and Immunology

www.aaaai.org

414-272-6071

555 East Wells Street, Suite 1100

Milwaukee, WI 53202-3823

American Celiac Society

www.americanceliacsociety.org

504-737-3293

P.O. Box 23455

New Orleans, LA 70183

Celiac Sprue Association, USA

www.csaceliacs.org
877-CSA-4CSA (-272-4272) or 402-558-0600
P.O. Box 31700
Omaha, NE 68131-0700

Children's PKU Network

www.pkunetwork.org/
3970 Via De La Valle, Suite 120
Del Mar, CA 92014

National Organization for Rare Disorders

www.rarediseases.org
800-999-6673 (voicemail) or 203-744-0100
P.O. Box 1968
Danbury, CT 06813-1968

Food Allergy and Anaphylaxis Network

www.foodallergy.org
800-929-4040
11781 Lee Jackson Highway, Suite 160
Fairfax, VA 22033-3309

Gluten Intolerance Group of North America

www.gluten.net
253-833-6655
31214 124th Avenue, S.E.
Auburn, WA 98092

Food Industry Associations

Almond Board of California
www.almondboard.com or www.AlmondsAreIn.com
888-597-8639 or 209-549-8262
1150 Ninth Street, Suite 1500
Modesto, CA 95354

American Egg Board
www.aeb.org or www.incredibleegg.org
www.eggsafety.org
847-296-7043 or 404-367-2761 (egg safety center)
1460 Renaissance Drive
Park Ridge, IL 60068

California Kiwi Fruit Commission
www.kiwifruit.org
916-441-0678
1521 I Street
Sacramento, CA 95814

California Olive Oil Council
www.cooc.com/
888-718-9830
P.O. Box 7520
Berkeley, CA 94707-0520

California Strawberry Commission
www.calstrawberry.com
831-724-1301
P.O. Box 269
Watsonville, CA 95077

California Table Grape Commission

www.grapesfromcalifornia.com

559-447-8350

392 West Fallbrook, Suite 101

Fresno, CA 93711

Calorie Control Council

www.caloriecontrol.org or *www.caloriescount.com*

404-252-3663

1100 Johnson Ferry Road, Suite 300

Atlanta, GA 30342

Dairy Management, Inc.

www.dairyinfo.com

800-853-2479 or 847-803-2000

O'Hare International Center

10255 West Higgins Road, Suite 900

Rosemont, IL 60018-5616

Distilled Spirits Council of the US

www.discus.org

202-628-3544

1250 Eye Street NW, Suite 400

Washington, D.C. 20005

Dole Food Company

www.dole.com

800-356-3111

P.O. Box 5700

Thousand Oaks, CA 91359-5700

Flax Council of Canada

www.flaxcouncil.ca

204-982-2115

465-167 Lombard Avenue

Winnipeg, MB

Canada R3B0T6

Florida Department of Citrus

www.floridajuice.com

863-537-3999

P.O. Box 9010

Bartow, FL 33831

Food Marketing Institute

www.fmi.org

202-452-8444

2345 Crystal Drive, Suite 800

Arlington, VA 22202

Infant Formula Council

www.infantformula.org

404-252-3663

110 Johnson Ferry Road, Suite 300

Atlanta, GA 30342

International Bottled Water Association

www.bottledwater.org

800-WATER-11 (-928-3711) or 703-683-5213

1700 Diagonal Road, Suite 650

Alexandria, VA 22314

International Food Information Council (IFIC)

www.ific.org

202-296-6540

1100 Connecticut Avenue, NW, Suite 430

Washington, D.C. 20036

National Cattlemen's Beef Association

www.beef.org

303-694-0305

9110 East Nichols Avenue #300

Centennial, CO 80112

National Chicken Council

www.nationalchickencouncil.com or *www.eatchicken.com*

202-296-2622

1015 15th Street, NW, Suite 930

Washington, D.C. 20005-2622

National Coffee Association

www.ncausa.org

212-766-4007

45 Broadway, Suite 1140

New York, NY 10006

National Dairy Council

www.nationaldairycouncil.org

916-263-3560

Dairy Council of California

1101 National Drive, Suite B

Sacramento, CA 95834

National Fisheries Institute, Inc.

www.aboutseafood.com/
703-524-8880
1901 North Fort Myer Drive, Suite 700
Arlington, VA 22209

National Pasta Association

www.ilovepasta.org
202-637-5888
750 National Press Building
529 14th Street, NW
Washington, D.C. 20045

National Potato Promotion Board

www.potatohelp.com
303-369-7783
U.S. Potato Board
7555 East Hampden Avenue, Suite 412
Denver, CO 80231

National Pork Producers Council

www.nppc.org
202-347-3600
122 C Street, NW, Suite 875
Washington, D.C. 20001

National Restaurant Association

www.restaurant.org/
800-424-5156 or 202-331-5900
1200 17th Street, NW
Washington, D.C. 20036-3097

The Peanut Institute

www.peanut-institute.org
888-8-PEANUT (-873-2688)
P.O. Box 70157
Albany, GA 31707

National Turkey Federation

www.turkeyfed.org or *www.eatturkey.com*
202-898-0100
1225 New York Avenue, NW, Suite 400
Washington, D.C. 20005

Oregon Dairy Center/Nutrition Education Services

www.oregondairycouncil.org
503-229-5033
10505 SW Barbur Boulevard
Portland, OR 97219

Pear Bureau Northwest

www.usapears.org
503-652-9720
4382 SE International Way, Suite A
Milwaukie, OR 97222

Produce for Better Health Foundation

www.fruitsandveggiesmorematters.org/
888-391-2100 or 302-235-2329
7465 Lancaster Pike, Suite J, 2nd Floor
Hockessin, DE 19707

Produce Marketing Association
www.pma.com
302-738-7100
P.O. Box 6036
Newark, DE 19714-6026

Snack Food Association
www.sfa.org
800-628-1334 or 703-836-4500
1600 Wilson Boulevard, Suite 650
Arlington, VA 22209

The Sugar Association, Inc.
www.sugar.org
202-785-1122
1300 L Street, NW, Suite 1001
Washington, D.C. 20005

The Tea Association of the U.S.A.
www.teausa.org
212-986-9415
362 Fifth Avenue, Suite 801
New York, NY 10001

United Fresh Produce Association
www.unitedfresh.org
202-303-3400
1901 Pennsylvania Avenue, NW, Suite 1100
Washington, D.C. 20006

United Soybean Board
www.soybean.org
800-989-8721
16305 Swingley Ridge Road, Suite 150
Chesterfield, MO 63017

USA Rice Federation

www.usarice.com
703-236-2300
4301 North Fairfax Drive, Suite 425
Arlington, VA 22203

U.S. Dry Bean Council

www.americanbean.com
360-277-0112
P.O. Box 550
Grapeview, WA 98546

Washington State Apple Commission

www.bestapples.com
509-663-9600
P.O. Box 18
Wenatchee, WA 98807

Washington State Fruit Commission/Northwest Cherries

www.nwcherries.com
509-453-4837
105 South 18th Street, Suite 205
Yakima, WA 98901

Wheat Foods Council

www.wheatfoods.org
970-626-9828
51D Red Fox Lane
Ridgway, Co 81432

Food Safety, Labeling, and Advertising

American Association of Poison Control Centers

www.aapcc.org

National hotline to local centers:

800-222-1222

Center for Nutrition Policy and Promotion

www.usda.gov/cnpp

703-305-7600

U.S. Department of Agriculture

3101 Park Center Drive, 10th Floor

Alexandria, VA 22302-1594

American Egg Board

www.aeb.org or *www.incredibleegg.org*

www.eggsafety.org

847-296-7043 or 404-367-2761 (egg safety center)

1460 Renaissance Drive

Park Ridge, IL 60068

Center for Food Safety and Applied Nutrition

www.fda.gov/Food/default.htm

888-SAFE-FOOD (723-3366)

CFSAN Outreach and Information Center

Food and Drug Administration

5100 Paint Branch Parkway

College Park, MD 20740

MEDWatch Program

www.fda.gov/MedWatch

800-FDA-1088 (-332-1088)

MedWatch

5600 Fishers Lane

Rockville, MD 20857

Federal Trade Commission (FTC)

www.ftc.gov

877-FTC-HELP (-382-4357) or 202-326-2222

600 Pennsylvania Avenue, NW, Room 130

Washington, D.C. 20580

Food and Drug Administration (FDA)

www.fda.gov

888-INFO-FDA (-463-6332)

Consumer Information Office

10903 New Hampshire Ave.

Silver Spring, MD 20993-0002

Food Safety and Inspection Service

www.fsis.usda.gov/

http://www.fsis.usda.gov/PDF/Kitchen_Companion.pdf

U.S. Department of Agriculture

1400 Independence Avenue, SW

Washington, D.C. 20250-3700

888-MP-Hotline (-674-6854) (USDA's Meat and Poultry Hotline)

International Food Information Council

www.foodinsight.org/

202-296-6540

1100 Connecticut Avenue, NW, Suite 430

Washington, D.C. 20036

Iowa State Extension

www.extension.iastate.edu/foodsafety
Food Safety Project Director
Iowa State University
Ames, IA, 50011-112

National Lead Information Center

www.epa.gov/lead
800-424-LEAD (-5323)
422 South Clinton Avenue
Rochester, NY 14620

U.S. Environmental Protection Agency

www.epa.gov
202-564-4700
Safe Drinking Water Hotline:
800-426-4791 *www.epa.gov/safewater*
Ariel Rios Building
1200 Pennsylvania Avenue, NW
Washington, D.C. 20460

U.S. Government

www.foodsafety.gov
U.S. Department of Health and Human Services
200 Independence Avenue, S.W.
Washington, D.C. 20201

Food Technology/Biotechnology

International Life Sciences Institute

www.ilsi.org

202-659-0074

1156 15th Street, NW, Suite 200

Washington, D.C. 20005

Office of Biotechnology Activities

http://oba.od.nih.gov/oba/

301-496-9838

National Institutes of Health

6705 Rockledge Drive, Suite 750

MSC 7985

Bethesda, MD 20892-7985

General Health Resources and Disease Prevention/Treatment

Alcoholism

Al-Anon/Alateen

http://www.al-anon.alateen.org (for information and meeting locations)

888-425-2666 or 888-4AL-ANON (425-2666)

Al-Anon Family Group Headquarters, Inc.

1600 Corporate Landing Parkway

Virginia Beach, VA 23454-5617

Alcoholics Anonymous

http://www.aa.org (for information and meeting locations)

212-870-3400

A.A. World Services, Inc., 11th Fl.

475 Riverside Drive at West 120th St.

New York, NY 10115

National Council on Alcoholism and Drug Dependence

www.ncadd.org

800-622-2255 or HOPE LINE:

800-NCA-CALL (622-2255) or 212-269-7797

244 East 58th Street, 4th Floor

New York, NY 10022

Substance Abuse & Mental Health Services Administration

http://ncadi.samhsa.gov/ or *www.samhsa.gov/shin/* (for publications)

800-729-6686 or 877-SAMHSA-7 (726-4727)

SAMHSA's Health Information Network

P.O. Box 2345

Rockville, MD 20847-2345

Cancer

American Cancer Society

www.cancer.org

800-227-2345 or 404-320-3333

250 Williams Street

Atlanta, GA 30303

American Institute for Cancer Research

www.aicr.org

800-843-8114 or 202-328-7744

1759 R Street, NW

Washington, D.C. 20009

National Cancer Institute

www.cancer.gov

800-4-CANCER (-422-6237) or 301-435-3848

NCI Office of Communications and Education

Public Inquiries Office

6116 Executive Boulevard, Suite 300

Bethesda, MD 20892-8322

Cardiovascular (Heart) Disease

American Heart Association

www.americanheart.org

800-AHA-USA1 (-242-8721)

7272 Greenville Avenue

Dallas, TX 75231-4596

National National Heart, Lung, and Blood Institute

www.nhlbi.nih.gov

301-592-8573

NHLBI Health Information Center

P.O. Box 30105

Bethesda, MD 20824-0105

Diabetes

American Diabetes Association

www.diabetes.org

800-DIABETES (-342-2383) or 703-549-1500

Center for Information

1701 North Beauregard Street

Alexandria, VA 22311

Joslin Diabetes Center

www.joslin.org

800-567-5461 or 617-732-2400

Nutrition Services

One Joslin Place

Boston, MA 02215

Juvenile Diabetes Research Foundation International

www.jdrf.org

800-JDF-CURE (-533-2873) or 212-785-9500

26 Broadway, 14th Floor

New York, NY 10004

National Diabetes Information Clearinghouse

http://diabetes.niddk.nih.gov/

800-860-8747

1 Information Way

Bethesda, MD 20892-3560

National Institute of Diabetes and Digestive and Kidney Diseases

www2.niddk.nih.gov/

301-496-3583

Office of Communications & Public Liaison, NIDDK, NIH

Building 31, Room 9A06

31 Center Drive, MSC 2560

Bethesda, MD 20892-2560

Digestive Disease

Digestive Disease National Coalition

www.ddnc.org

202-544-7497

507 Capitol Court NE, Suite 200

Washington, D.C. 20002

National Digestive Diseases Information Clearinghouse

http://digestive.niddk.nih.gov/

800-891-5389 or 301-654-3810

2 Information Way

Bethesda, MD 20892-3570

Eating Disorders

Eating Disorder Referral and Information Center

www.edreferral.com

**National Association of Anorexia Nervosa
and Associated Disorders**

www.anad.org/

ANAD Helpline 630-577-1330

P.O. Box 640

Naperville, IL 60566

National Eating Disorders Organization

www.nationaleatingdisorders.org/

206-382-3587

603 Stewart Street, Suite 803

Seattle, WA 98101

General

American Academy of Family Physicians
www.aafp.org
800-274-2237 or 913-906-6000
11400 Tomahawk Creek Parkway
Leawood, KS 66211-2672

American Health Foundation
www.americanhealthfoundation.com/
561-361-9091
P.O. Box 1172
Boca Raton, FL 33429

American Medical Association
www.ama-assn.org
800-621-8335 or 312-464-5000
515 North State Street
Chicago, IL 60654

American Public Health Association
www.apha.org
202-777-2742 (-777-APHA)
800 I street, NW
Washington, D.C. 20001-3710

C.D.C.'s National Prevention Information Network
www.cdcnpin.org/
800-458-5231 or 404-679-3860
or 800-CDC-INFO (-232-4636)(for printed materials requests)
Clearinghouse for HIV/AIDs, STDs, and TB material
P.O. Box 6003
Rockville, MD 20849-6003

Centers for Disease Control and Prevention

www.cdc.gov

800-CDC-INFO (-232-4636) or 404-639-3311

1600 Clifton Road NE

Atlanta, GA 30333

Congress for National Health

www.nationalwellness.org

715-342-2969

National Wellness Institute

P.O. Box 827

Stevens Point, WI 54481-0827

Minority Health Resource Center

http://minorityhealth.hhs.gov/

800-444-6472

Office of Minority Health

Resource Center

P.O. Box 37337

Washington, D.C. 20013-7337

National Center for Health Statistics

www.cdc.gov/nchs

800-232-4636 (-CDC-INFO)

3311 Toledo Road

Hyattsville, MD 20782

National Health Information Center

www.health.gov/nhic or *www.healthfinder.gov*

800-336-4797 or 301-565-4167

P.O. Box 1133

Washington, D.C. 20013-1133

Toll-free health information:

www.health.gov/nhic/pubs/2010tollfreenumbers/tollfreenumbers1.htm

Federal health information and clearinghouses:

www.health.gov/nhic/pubs/2010clearinghouses/clearinghouses.htm

National Institutes of Health

http://health.nih.gov/

301-496-4000

9000 Rockville Pike

Bethesda, MD 20892

U.S. Department of Health and Human Services

www.hhs.gov or

www.healthcare.gov (for information on healthcare reform)

877-696-6775 (HHS hotline)

200 Independence Avenue, SW

Washington, D.C. 20201

Oral Health

American Dental Association

www.ada.org

312-440-2500

211 East Chicago Avenue

Chicago, IL 60611-2678

Osteoporosis

National Osteoporosis Foundation
www.nof.org
800-231-4222 or 202-223-2226
1150 17th Street NW, Suite 850
Washington, D.C. 20036

Weight

Healthy Weight Network
www.healthyweight.net
701-567-2646
402 South 14th Street
Hettinger, ND 58639

Overeaters Anonymous
www.oa.org/
505-891-2664
P.O. Box 44020
Rio Rancho, New Mexico 87174-4020

Shape Up America
www.shapeup.org
PO Box 149
506 Brackett Creek Road
Clyde Park, MT 59018

Gardening and Farming

California Foundation for Agriculture in the Classroom
www.cfaitc.org
916-561-5625
2300 River Plaza Drive
Sacramento, CA 95833-3293

Farm to School Program
www.fns.usda.gov/cnd/F2S/
Food & Nutrition Service
3101 Park Center Drive
Alexandria, VA 22302

National Gardening Association
www.garden.org/
800-538-7476 or 802-863-5251
National Gardening Association
1100 Dorset Street
South Burlington, VT 05403

North Carolina State University
http://www.cals.ncsu.edu/hort_sci/
919-515-3131 or 252-237-0111
Department of Horticultural Science
2721 Founders Drive
Raleigh, NC 27695

Washington State University
www.pierce.wsu.edu
253-798-7180
WSU Pierce County Extension
3602 Pacific Avenue, Suite B
Tacoma, WA 98418-7920

Health Fraud

National Council Against Health Fraud
www.ncahf.org
919-533-6009

Maternal, Infant, Child, and Pediatric Nutrition

Action for Healthy Kids
www.actionforhealthykids.org
800-416-1849
4711 Golf Road, Suite 625
Skokie, IL 60076

American Academy of Pediatrics
www.aap.org
847-434-4000
141 Northwest Point Boulevard
Elk Grove Village, IL 60007-1098

School Nutrition Association
www.schoolnutrition.org
800-877-8822 or 301-686-3100
School Nutrition Association
120 Waterfront Street, Suite 300
National Harbor, MD 20745

Nutrition Explorations

www.nutritionexplorations.org

847-803-2000

National Dairy Council

10255 West Higgins Road, Suite 900

Rosemont, IL 60018-5616

Nutrition for Kids

www.nutritionforkids.com

503-524-9318

24 Carrot Press

P.O. Box 23546

Portland, OR 97281-3546

University of Nebraska

http://lancaster.unl.edu/food/

402-441-7180

UNL Lincoln Extension in Lancaster County

444 Cherrycreek Road, Suite A

Lincoln, NE 68528

Health Resources and Services Administration

http://mchb.hrsa.gov/about/default.htm

Maternal and Child Health Bureau

Parklawn Building Room 18-05

5600 Fishers Lane, Rockville, MD 20857

La Leche League International

www.llli.org/

800-LA-LECHE (800-525-3243) or 847-519-7730

957 North Plumgrove Road

Schaumburg, IL 60173

USDA/ARS Children's Nutrition Research Center

www.bcm.tmc.edu/cnrc

713-798-6767

Baylor College of Medicine

One Baylor Plaza

Houston, TX 77030

Nutrition and Aging

American Association of Retired Persons

www.aarp.org

888-OUR-AARP(-687-2277)or 202-243-3525

601 E Street, NW

Washington, D.C. 20049

National Association of Area Agencies on Aging

www.n4a.org

202-872-0888

1730 Rhode Island Ave, NW, Suite 1200

Washington, D.C. 20036

Elder Care Locator

www.eldercare.gov/

800-677-1116

National Institute on Aging Information Office

www.nih.gov/nia

301-496-1752

Building 31, Room 5C27

31 Center Drive, MSC 2292

Bethesda, MD 20892

Nutrition Newsletters

Consumer Reports on Health

www.consumerreports.org/health

800-274-7596 or 914-378-2300

101 Truman Avenue

Yonkers, NY 10703

Environmental Nutrition

www.environmentalnutrition.com

800-424-7887

P.O. Box 5656

Norwalk, CT 06856-5656

Communicating Food for Health Newsletter

http://communicatingfoodforhealth.com/

954-385-5328 (info)

P.O. Box 266498

Weston, FL 33326

Food & Fitness Advisor

www.foodandfitnessadvisor.com

800-829-2505

The Center for Women's Health

Weill Medical College of Cornell University

P.O. Box 420235

Palm Coast, FL 32142-0235

Mayo Clinic Health Letter

www.mayohealth.org

800-333-9037

Subscription Services

P.O. Box 9302

Big Sandy, TX 75755

Tufts University Health and Nutrition Letter

www.tuftshealthletter.com

800-274-7581

Subscription Services

P.O. Box 8517

Big Sandy, TX 75755

University of California, Berkeley Wellness Letter

www.berkeleywellness.com/

800-829-9170

Subscription Department

P.O. Box 420235

Palm Coast, FL 32142-0235

U.S. Government Printing Office

http://www.gpoaccess.gov

866-512-1800 or 202-512-1800

Superintendent of Documents

732 North Capitol Street, NW

Washington, D.C. 20401

Nutrition Sites For Kids:

Body and Mind

www.bam.gov

Dole Super Kids

www.dole.com/#/superkids

Kidnetic

www.kidnetic.com

Kids Health

www.kidshealth.org/kid

Let's Move

www.letsmove.gov/eat-healthy

Science 4 Kids (Agricultural Research Service)

www.ars.usda.gov/is/kids/

Smart-Mouth

www.smart-mouth.org

School Foodservice

Healthy Meals Resource System

http://healthymeals.nal.usda.gov

301-504-6366

Food And Nutrition Information Center

National Agriculture Library

10301 Baltimore Boulevard, Room 105

Beltsville, MD 20705-2351

Division of Adolescent and School Health (DASH)

www.cdc.gov/HealthyYouth/

800-CDC-INFO (-232-4636)

Centers for Disease Control and Prevention

Healthy Schools Healthy Youth Program

1600 Clifton Road

Atlanta, GA 30333

National Food Service Management Institute

www.olemiss.edu/depts/nfsmi

800-321-3054 or 662-915-7658

The University of Mississippi

6 Jeanette Phillips Drive

P.O. Drawer 188

University, MS 38677-0188

School Nutrition Association

www.schoolnutrition.org

703-739-3900

120 Waterfront Street, Suite 300

National Harbor, MD 20745

Team Nutrition

www.fns.usda.gov/tn

703-305-1624

USDA's Team Nutrition

3101 Park Center Drive, Room 632

Alexandria, VA 22302

Sports Nutrition
and Physical Activity

American Alliance for Health, Physical Education,

Recreation, and Dance

www.aahperd.org

800-213-7193 or 703-476-3400

1900 Association Drive

Reston, VA 20191-1598

American College of Sports Medicine

www.acsm.org

317-637-9200

P.O. Box 1440

Indianapolis, IN 46206-1440

American Council on Exercise

www.acefitness.org/

800-825-3636 or 858-576-6582

4851 Paramount Drive

San Diego, CA 92123

American Running Association

www.americanrunning.org

800-776-ARFA (-2732 or 301-913-9517

4405 East-West Highway, Suite 405

Bethesda, MD 20814

Center for Weight and Health

http://cwh.berkeley.edu/

510-642-2915

University of California, Berkeley

3 Giannini Hall

Berkeley, CA 94720-3100

Lifelong Fitness Alliance

www.lifelongfitnessalliance.org

650-361-8282

2682 Middlefield Road, Suite Z

Redwood City, CA 94063

International Society for Sports Nutrition

www.sportsnutritionsociety.org
866-740-4776
600 Pembrook Drive
Woodland Park, CO 80863

President's Council on Fitness, Sports, and Nutrition

www.fitness.gov/ and *www.letsmove.gov/get-active*
240-276-9567
1101 Wootton Parkway, Suite 560
Rockville, MD 20852

President's Fitness Challenge

www.presidentschallenge.org
800-258-8146
501 North Morton, Suite 203
Bloomington, IN 47404

Women's Sports Foundation

www.womenssportsfoundation.org/
800-227-3988 or 516-542-4700
National Office
Eisenhower Park
1899 Hempstead Turnpike, Suite 400
East Meadow, NY 11554

YMCA of the USA

www.ymca.net/
800-USA-YMCA (-872-9622) or 312-977-0031
101 North Wacker Drive
Chicago, IL 60606

Vegetarian Eating

North American Vegetarian Society
www.navs-online.org
518-568-7970
P.O. Box 72
Dolgeville, NY 13329

Vegetarian Resource Group
www.vrg.org
410-366-VEGE (-8343)
P.O. Box 1463
Baltimore, MD 21203

Fitness and Health

Clark, N. *Nancy Clark's Sports Nutrition Guidebook,* 4th ed. Champaign, IL: Human Kinetics Publishing; 2008.

Coleman E, Steen SN. *The Ultimate Sports Nutrition Book,* 2nd ed. Palo Alto, CA: Bull Publishing; 2000.

Jennings DS, Steen SN. *Play Hard, Eat Right: A Parent's Guide to Sports Nutrition for Children,* Minnetonka, MN: Wiley Publishing, 1995.

General Reference

Betty Crocker Editors. *Betty Crocker Cookbook: Everything You Need to Know to Cook Today,* 10th ed. Hoboken, NJ: Wiley Publishing; 2005.

Duyff RL. *American Dietetic Association Complete Food and Nutrition Guide,* 3rd ed. Hoboken, NJ: Wiley Publishing, 2006.

Evers, CL. *How to Teach Nutrition to Kids,* 3rd ed. Portland, OR: 24 Carrot Press; 2006.

Patten E, Lyons K. *Healthy Foods from Healthy Soils.* Gardiner, ME: Tillbury House Publishers; 2003.

.

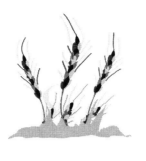

INDEX

Walking. *See* Activity

Water, 12, 20-28, 37, 86, 95, 98, 120-125
        exercise and, 122-127
        functions of, 12, 25-27, 98, 102, 123-124
        health benefits of, 12, 25-27, 98, 102, 123-124

Web sites, 254-292. *See also* Resource section
        ChooseMyPlate, 260
        food safety related, 166, 270-272

Weight, body, 68-69, 101-135, 287-288
        body mass index (BMI) and, 115-117
        behavior change and, 15, 129-133
        health risk and, 9, 21, 46, 67, 114
        physical activity and, 121-126, 289-292
        reduction tips, 76, 95, 112-135

Whole grains. *See* Grains

Wine, 81-82
        grape juice compared to, 82
        resveratrol in, 81

Yams, Baked, 216

Zucchini Bread, Reduced Fat, 217-218